Sports Medicine Statistics

Editors

JOE M. HART
STEPHEN R. THOMPSON

CLINICS IN SPORTS MEDICINE

www.sportsmed.theclinics.com

Consulting Editor
MARK D. MILLER

July 2018 • Volume 37 • Number 3

ELSEVIER

1600 John F. Kennedy Boulevard • Suite 1800 • Philadelphia, Pennsylvania, 19103-2899

http://www.theclinics.com

CLINICS IN SPORTS MEDICINE Volume 37, Number 3
July 2018 ISSN 0278-5919, ISBN-13: 978-0-323-61291-3

Editor: Lauren Boyle
Developmental Editor: Donald Mumford

Clinics in Sports Medicine (ISSN 0278-5919) is published quarterly by Elsevier Inc., 360 Park Avenue South, New York, NY 10010-1710. Months of issue are January, April, July, and October. Business and Editorial Offices: 1600 John F. Kennedy Blvd., Ste. 1800, Philadelphia, PA 19103-2899. Customer Service Office: 3251 Riverport Lane, Maryland Heights, MO 63043. Periodicals postage paid at New York, NY and additional mailing offices. Subscription prices are $357.00 per year (US individuals), $664.00 per year (US institutions), $100.00 per year (US students), $405.00 per year (Canadian individuals), $820.00 per year (Canadian institutions), $235.00 (Canadian students), $475.00 per year (foreign individuals), $820.00 per year (foreign institutions), and $235.00 per year (foreign students). Foreign air speed delivery is included in all *Clinics* subscription prices. All prices are subject to change without notice. **POSTMASTER:** Send address changes to *Clinics in Sports Medicine*, Elsevier Health Sciences Division, Subscription Customer Service, 3251 Riverport Lane, Maryland Heights, MO 63043. Customer Service (orders, claims, online, change of address): Elsevier Health Sciences Division, Subscription Customer Service, 3251 Riverport Lane, Maryland Heights, MO 63043. **Tel: 1-800-654-2452 (U.S. and Canada); 314-447-8871 (outside U.S. and Canada). Fax: 314-447-8029. E-mail: journalscustomerservice-usa@elsevier.com (for print support); journalsonlinesupport-usa@ elsevier.com (for online support).**

Reprints. For copies of 100 or more of articles in this publication, please contact the Commercial Reprints Department, Elsevier Inc., 360 Park Avenue South, New York, NY 10010-1710. Tel.: 212-633-3874; Fax: 212-633-3820; E-mail: reprints@elsevier.com.

Clinics in Sports Medicine is covered in *MEDLINE/PubMed (Index Medicus) Current Contents/Clinical Medicine, Excerpta Medica,* and *ISI/Biomed.*

Contributors

CONSULTING EDITOR

MARK D. MILLER, MD
S. Ward Casscells Professor, Head, Department of Orthopaedic Surgery, Division of Sports Medicine, University of Virginia, Charlottesville, Virginia, USA; Team Physician, James Madison University, Director, Miller Review Course, Harrisonburg, Virginia, USA

EDITORS

JOE M. HART, PhD, ATC
Associate Professor, Kinesiology, Director of Clinical Research, Orthopaedic Surgery, University of Virginia, Charlottesville, Virginia, USA

STEPHEN R. THOMPSON, MD, MEd, FRCSC
Associate Professor of Sports Medicine, Eastern Maine Medical Center, University of Maine, Bangor, Maine, USA

AUTHORS

CHRISTY L. COLLINS, PhD
President, Datalys Center for Sports Injury Research and Prevention, Inc, Indianapolis, Indiana, USA

SAULO DELFINO BARBOZA, MSc
PhD Student, Amsterdam Collaboration on Health and Safety in Sports, Department of Public and Occupational Health, Amsterdam Public Health Research Institute, VU University Medical Center, Amsterdam, The Netherlands

ALEXANDRA B. GIL, PT, PhD
Assistant Professor, Department of Physical Therapy, University of Pittsburgh, Pittsburgh, Pennsylvania, USA

JAY HERTEL, PhD, ATC
Joe H. Gieck Professor of Sports Medicine, Departments of Kinesiology and Orthopaedic Surgery, University of Virginia, Charlottesville, Virginia, USA

MACKENZIE M. HERZOG, MPH
PhD Candidate, Department of Epidemiology, The University of North Carolina at Chapel Hill, Chapel Hill, North Carolina, USA; Epidemiologist, Real-World Evidence, IQVIA, Research Triangle Park, Durham, North Carolina, USA

JAMES J. IRRGANG, PT, PhD, ATC, FAPTA
Professor, Department of Physical Therapy, University of Pittsburgh, Pittsburgh, Pennsylvania, USA

MELISSA C. KAY, MS, LAT, ATC
Doctoral Candidate, Department of Exercise and Sport Science, Matthew Gfeller Sport-Related Traumatic Brain Injury Research Center, The University of North Carolina at Chapel Hill, Chapel Hill, North Carolina, USA

KRISTEN L. KUCERA, PhD, MSPH, LAT, ATC
Assistant Professor, Department of Exercise and Sport Science, Director National Center for Catastrophic Sports Injury Research, Matthew Gfeller Sport-Related Traumatic Brain Injury Research Center, The University of North Carolina at Chapel Hill, Chapel Hill, North Carolina, USA

MONICA R. LININGER, PhD, LAT, ATC
Assistant Professor, Department of Physical Therapy and Athletic Training, Athletic Training Education Program, Northern Arizona University, Flagstaff, Arizona, USA

NIV MAROM, MD
Department of Sports Medicine, Hospital for Special Surgery, New York, New York, USA

STEPHEN W. MARSHALL, PhD
Professor, Department of Epidemiology, The University of North Carolina at Chapel Hill, Director, Injury Prevention Research Center, Chapel Hill, North Carolina, USA

ROBERT G. MARX, MD
Department of Sports Medicine, Hospital for Special Surgery, New York, New York, USA

SARAH N. MORRIS, PhD
Biostatistician, Datalys Center for Sports Injury Research and Prevention, Inc, Indianapolis, Indiana, USA

SARA R. PIVA, PT, PhD
Associate Professor, Department of Physical Therapy, University of Pittsburgh, Pittsburgh, Pennsylvania, USA

ROLAND RÖSSLER, PhD
Amsterdam Collaboration on Health and Safety in Sports, Department of Public and Occupational Health, Amsterdam Public Health Research Institute, VU University Medical Center, Amsterdam, The Netherlands; Department of Sport, Exercise and Health, University of Basel, Basel, Switzerland

BRYAN L. RIEMANN, PhD, ATC, FNATA
Professor of Sports Medicine, Biodynamics and Human Performance Center, Georgia Southern University, Savannah, Georgia, USA

JOSEPH J. RUZBARSKY, MD
Department of Sports Medicine, Hospital for Special Surgery, New York, New York, USA

UJASH SHETH, MD, MSc
Division of Orthopaedic Surgery, University of Toronto, Toronto, Ontario, Canada

KURT P. SPINDLER, MD
Vice Chair of Research and Orthopaedic Surgeon, Orthopaedic Sports Medicine, Cleveland Clinic, Cleveland, Ohio, USA

JOSÉ F. VEGA, MA
Cleveland Clinic Lerner College of Medicine, Case Western Reserve University, Orthopaedic Sports Medicine, Cleveland Clinic, Cleveland, Ohio, USA

EVERT VERHAGEN, PhD
Amsterdam Collaboration on Health and Safety in Sports, Department of Public and Occupational Health, Amsterdam Public Health Research Institute, VU University Medical Center, Amsterdam, The Netherlands; Division of Exercise Science and Sports Medicine, University of Cape Town, Cape Town, South Africa

ERIN B. WASSERMAN, PhD
Director, NCAA Injury Prevention Program, Datalys Center for Sports Injury Research and Prevention, Inc, Indianapolis, Indiana, USA

DAVID WASSERSTEIN, MD, MSc, MPH, FRCSC
Assistant Professor, Division of Orthopaedic Surgery, Sunnybrook Health Sciences Centre, Division of Orthopaedic Surgery, University of Toronto, Toronto, Ontario, Canada

EVERT VERHAGEN, PhD
Amsterdam Collaboration on Health and Safety in Sports, Department of Public and Occupational Health, Amsterdam Public Health research Institute, VU University Medical Center, Amsterdam, The Netherlands; Division of Exercise Science and Sports Medicine, University of Cape Town, Cape Town, South Africa

ERIN E. WASSERMAN, PhD
Director, NCAA Injury Prevention Program, Datalys Center for Sports Injury Research and Prevention, Inc, Indianapolis, Indiana, USA

DAVID WASSERSTEIN, MD, MSc, MPH, FRCSC
Assistant Professor, Division of Orthopaedic Surgery, Sunnybrook Health Sciences Centre, Division of Orthopaedic Surgery, University of Toronto, Toronto, Ontario, Canada

Contents

> Understanding the results and statistics reported in original research re-
> mains a large challenge for many sports medicine practitioners and, in
> turn, may be among one of the biggest barriers to integrating research
> into sports medicine practice. This article provides minimal essentials a
> sports medicine practitioner needs to know about interpreting statistics
> and research results to facilitate the incorporation of the latest evidence
> into practice. Topics covered include the difference between statistical
> significance and clinical meaningfulness; effect sizes and confidence inter-
> vals; reliability statistics, including the minimal detectable difference and
> minimal important difference; and statistical power.

> Recently, the importance of statistics and analytics in sports has
> increased. This article describes measures of sports injury and fundamen-
> tals of sports injury research with a brief overview of some of the emerging
> measures of sports performance. The authors describe research study de-
> signs that can be used to identify risk factors for injury, injury surveillance
> programs, and common measures of injury risk and association. Finally,
> we describe measures of physical performance and training and consider-
> ations for using these measures. This article provides sports medicine cli-
> nicians with an understanding of current research measures and
> considerations for designing sports injury research studies.

> Mixed methods research is a relatively new approach in the field of sports
> medicine, where the benefits of qualitative and quantitative research are
> combined while offsetting the other's flaws. Despite its known and suc-
> cessful use in other populations, it has been used minimally in sports med-
> icine, including studies of the clinician perspective, concussion, and
> patient outcomes. Therefore, there is a need for this approach to be
> applied in other topic areas not easily addressed by one type of research
> approach in isolation, such as the retirement from sport, effects of and re-
> turn from injury, and catastrophic injury.

> There has been a dramatic increase in the use of large-scale health administrative databases to investigate clinical outcomes within sports medicine over the past few years. Although these data sets identify large numbers of patients, allowing for the investigation of regional trends, health care utilization, and outcomes of surgical intervention, they were not designed with the intention of answering clinical questions. Recognizing the methodological limitations associated with these databases is prudent to avoid propagating spurious conclusions. This article offers an overview of the administrative databases commonly used within the orthopedic sports medicine literature and provides key principles for their critical appraisal.

> The Multicenter Orthopaedic Outcomes Network (MOON) is a one of the largest prospective cohorts in orthopedic sports medicine. It comprises 17 fellowship-trained surgeons from 7 different institutions and has enrolled more than 4000 patients, with follow-up exceeding 80% at 2, 6, and 10 years postop. This article chronicles the development and execution of MOON, taking the reader on a journey that begins in 1991, with the dream of MOON, and continues until the present day, with the current state of MOON, including all of the trials and tribulations encountered along the way.

FORTHCOMING ISSUES

October 2018
Shoulder Arthritis in the Young and Active Patient
Stephen F. Brockmeier and
Brian C. Werner, *Editors*

January 2019
OrthoBiologics in Sports Medicine
Rachel M. Frank and Brian J. Cole, *Editors*

April 2009
Knee MLI
Bruce A. Levy and Benjamin Freychet, *Editors*

RECENT ISSUES

April 2018
Common Procedures—Common Problems
Mark D. Miller, *Editor*

January 2018
Controversies of the Anterolateral Complex of the Knee
Freddie H. Fu and Marcin Kowalczuk, *Editors*

October 2017
The Female Athlete
Siobhan M. Statuta, *Editor*

RELATED INTEREST

Physical Medicine and Rehabilitation Clinics, May 2016 (Volume 27, Issue 2)
Concussion in Sports
Scott R. Laker, *Editor*

THE CLINICS ARE AVAILABLE ONLINE!
Access your subscription at:
www.theclinics.com

Foreword

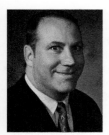

Mark D. Miller, MD
Consulting Editor

*A certain elementary training in statistical method is becoming as necessary for
everyone living in this world of today as reading and writing.*

—*H.G. Wells*

Some readers may ask, "After so many cool state-of-the-art issues that have been
published in *Clinics in Sports Medicine*, why did you pick such a boring topic for
this issue?" As much as I like the Mark Twain quote (which some attribute to
Benjamin Disraeli) provided in the preface to this issue, statistics is a necessary disci-
pline—especially in medicine; so sometimes we need to make sure that we know how
to interpret the science behind the research, not just show new and interesting
procedures.

Over the years, I have struggled to find dynamic and interesting lecturers on statistics and have failed more often than not. Luckily, I eventually chanced upon two who
have succeeded, Drs Joe Hart and Steve Thompson. Both Joe and Steve have given
this challenging lecture topic at the Miller Review Course, and against all odds (statistically speaking), delivered well-reviewed and well-appreciated lectures. That's why I
asked them to team up and provide our readership some elementary training in statistical methods.

Like all issues of *Clinics in Sports Medicine*, this represents a complete and thorough
review of the "significant" issues of this topic. It includes statistical and analytical principles, mixed model designs, prevention and interpretation studies, graph interpretation, quality and outcome reporting, and guidelines for interpreting administrative
databases, and concludes with a "lessons-learned" discussion from the MOON group.
For those who are not familiar with this last topic, suffice it to say that the MOON group,
led by Dr Kurt Spindler, was the first "extraterrestrial" named sports medicine group to
report multicenter outcome data and continues to do so at virtually every orthopedic
sports medicine meeting and in every journal published. It is the model design for

Clin Sports Med 37 (2018) xi–xii
https://doi.org/10.1016/j.csm.2018.05.001
0278-5919/18/© 2018 Published by Elsevier Inc.

reporting important outcome data. This is a great issue of *Clinics in Sports Medicine*. Thanks to Joe Hart and Steve Thompson for putting together such an excellent treatise on statistics in sports medicine.

Thanks!

Mark D. Miller, MD
Division of Sports Medicine
Department of Orthopaedic Surgery
University of Virginia
James Madison University Director
400 Ray C. Hunt Drive, Suite 330
Charlottesville, VA 22908-0159, USA

E-mail address:
mdm3p@virginia.edu

Preface

Sports Medicine Statistics

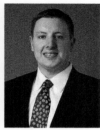

Joe M. Hart, PhD, ATC   Stephen R. Thompson, MD, MEd, FRCSC
Editors

As Mark Twain so famously wrote, there are lies, damn lies, and statistics. In today's age with the massive proliferation of open access, as well as predatory journals, there has never been more access to scholarly manuscripts. Consequently, it has become incumbent upon the reader to approach each study with increasing scrutiny and to question the veracity of the findings.

In addition, the research is becoming increasingly complex. A recent study was published with the subheading of "A Meta-Analysis of Randomized Controlled Trials and Systematic Review of Overlapping Systematic Reviews." A review of reviews? Dizzying!

In this present issue, we hope to present to the reader a primer on how sports medicine research and statistics are evolving into the third decade of the twenty-first century. It is our sincere hope that this provides guidance for consumers of medical research. Like any accomplished medical practitioner, successful practice relies on not only the available tools but also the manner in which they are used. Statistics are like tools in a toolbox that when used correctly can lead to discovery and innovation, however, when used incorrectly, can be misleading and potentially dangerous. In this issue, we have invited top scholars in statistics, clinical research design, mixed methodology, sports analytics, and injury prevention to provide a primer in clinical research statistics. The articles in this issue of *Clinics in Sports Medicine* provide an outstanding overview of contemporary approaches to research design, analysis, and data presentation that are geared toward sports medicine professionals. To lead off the issue, Dr Bryan Riemann and Dr Erin Wasserman provide outstanding fundamental reviews of biostatistics and data analytics for the sports medicine professional, after which are articles that provide statistical reviews in injury prevention, mixed model research designs, and clinical trials. Then, Dr Jay Hertel provides an excellent overview of contemporary and novel approaches to presenting data that will truly make readers consider the best approach to data visualization. These articles provide invaluable

Clin Sports Med 37 (2018) xiii–xiv
https://doi.org/10.1016/j.csm.2018.04.002
0278-5919/18/© 2018 Published by Elsevier Inc.   **sportsmed.theclinics.com**

resources for interpretation and critical review of sports medicine research to enable decision making and evidence-based practice.

Following this, we are delighted to have one of the very rare individuals to have an eponymous outcome measure, Dr Bob Marx, and his colleagues, Dr Ruzbarsky and Dr Maron, who provide an outstanding review of the psychometric properties of patient-reported outcome measures as applicable to sports medicine.

Next, Dr Wasserstein, from the University of Toronto, provides an excellent overview of how administrative databases are employed in sports medicine research. Last, one of the most influential multicenter collaborations in sports medicine has been the Multicenter Orthopedic Outcomes Network (MOON) group. Owing to their prolific output, it is important to understand how this group came about, how their research cohorts have been developed, and what lessons they have learned throughout the course of their almost 30-year history. Its founding member, Dr Kurt Spindler from the Cleveland Clinic, has provided an excellent overview of his lessons from "The MOON."

We are grateful to Dr Miller, the consulting editor, for asking us to pair up and to be able to combine the perspectives of a practicing sports medicine orthopedic surgeon alongside a full-time PhD researcher in orthopedic sports medicine.

Joe M. Hart, PhD, ATC
Kinesiology
Clinical Research, Orthopaedic Surgery
University of Virginia
Charlottesville, VA 22904, USA

Stephen R. Thompson, MD, MEd, FRCSC
Eastern Maine Medical Center
University of Maine
Bangor, ME 04401, USA

E-mail addresses:
joehart@virginia.edu (J.M. Hart)
theskip@gmail.com (S.R. Thompson)

Principles of Statistics
What the Sports Medicine Professional Needs to Know

Bryan L. Riemann, PhD, ATC, FNATA[a],*,
Monica R. Lininger, PhD, LAT, ATC[b]

KEYWORDS

- Clinical meaningfulness • P values • Data interpretation • Confidence intervals
- Effect sizes • Statistical power • Minimal detectable difference
- Minimal important difference

KEY POINTS

- Statistical significance reflects the influence of chance on the outcome, whereas clinical meaningfulness reflects the degree to which the study results reported are relevant to sports medicine practice.
- When statistically significant differences are revealed, confidence intervals and effect sizes can be used to enhance the practical interpretation of the research results.
- Absolute reliability characteristics, such as the minimal detectable change, determine the extent of error around a measurement and, when coupled with an appropriate minimal important difference estimate, can assist in triangulating clinically meaningful changes in patients undergoing treatment.
- In the circumstance of nonstatistically significant results, evaluation needs to occur to determine if the study had adequate statistical power prior to concluding no difference or association exists.

Along with many disciplines in medicine and allied health, the evidence-based practice (EBP) movement has prompted practitioners in the field of sports medicine to have a better competency in understanding research. As new procedures, methods, and understanding are studied with the results presented in research studies, practicing sports medicine professionals are faced with evaluating both statistically significant and clinically meaningful benefit along with whether the results are pertinent to their patients. Unquestionably, interpreting statistical findings as part of the research

Disclosure Statement: No conflicts of interest pertaining to this work.
[a] Sports Medicine, Biodynamics and Human Performance Center, Georgia Southern University, 11935 Abercorn Street, Savannah, GA 31419, USA; [b] Physical Therapy and Athletic Training, Athletic Training Education Program, Northern Arizona University, PO Box 15094, Flagstaff, AZ 86011, USA
* Corresponding author.
E-mail address: briemann@georgiasouthern.edu

Clin Sports Med 37 (2018) 375–386
https://doi.org/10.1016/j.csm.2018.03.004
0278-5919/18/© 2018 Elsevier Inc. All rights reserved.

evaluation process can be a daunting challenge for many practitioners. Few practitioners enter a field, such as sports medicine, wanting to develop and possess an extensive expertise in statistics. Fortunately, once command over some of the nomenclature and few key concepts, along with understanding the more common statistical procedures, is attained, practitioners can often begin to evaluate research. The purpose of this article is to provide minimal essentials a sports medicine professional needs to know about interpreting statistics and research results to facilitate the incorporation of the latest evidence into practice. Topics covered include the difference between statistical significance and clinical meaningfulness; effect sizes and confidence intervals; reliability statistics, including the minimal detectable difference (MDD) and minimal important difference (MID); and statistical power. To begin the discussion, some of the common research and statistical terms are presented in **Table 1**.

ROLE OF STATISTICS IN THE RESEARCH PROCESS

Research, the process of acquiring new knowledge through systematic data collection procedures followed by controlled and critical analysis of the data, is one of the foundations of EBP. It is the analysis of data part of this definition for which statistics become necessary. One of the first tasks after data are collected is to summarize the data so they may be reduced into smaller and more interpretable chunks. Descriptive statistics are those indicators that are used to portray the data in more interpretable chunks. The challenge is that no single descriptive statistic can represent an entire data set as a single value. For example, the mean change in range of motion can be described for 2 groups as 10°; however, closer inspection of the individual participants may yield a different perspective (**Table 2**). Thus, at minimum, the optimal approach is to provide some indicator of the data set center and the extent of variation around the center. The measurement scale of the data dictates the appropriate descriptive statistics to use (**Table 3**).

In research, it is not feasible to study all members of a defined population. Because research involves selecting a sample from a target population, assumptions and hypotheses must be examined to determine whether the obtained results are tenable or if they could have simply occurred due to chance. Additionally, a researcher often wants to generalize or make predictions about the population from which a sample was obtained. A population is defined as all individuals who meet the inclusion and exclusion criteria for a specific study. When a sample is drawn from the population, sampling error is likely incurred because it is probable that the sample does not perfectly represent (ie, duplicate) a population. Thus, estimates about what exists in the entire population based on the sample differ from the true reality. The magnitude of sampling error is attempted to be decreased through using optimal research design elements, including random sampling and random allocation (assignment), sufficiently sized samples, and reliable outcome measures. Despite the efforts to decrease sampling error, some uncertainty always exists; the challenge for researchers and practitioners alike is how to evaluate whether the difference/relationship results are real versus the likelihood that they occurred based on chance (ie, sampling error). By providing a *P* value, inferential statistics attempt to provide some indication regarding the extent to which chance might explain the results.

INTERPRETING *P* VALUES

Interpretation of the resulting *P* values from inferential statistics is an area of frequent confusion. Two perspectives on using *P* values have been described, significance testing and hypothesis testing. Over the years the 2 perspectives have often become

Table 1
Commonly used terms in research and statistics

Term	Definition
Population	The target population is all participants who meet a specified set of inclusion and exclusion criteria. In practice, it is not possible to have access to all persons meeting the criteria; the accessible population is the portion of the target population that the researcher has access from which to select participants.
Sample	The selected sample is the group of persons selected from the accessible population who are asked to participate in the study. The actual sample is the group of participants who complete the study and whose data is used for analysis.
Random sampling	The selection of selecting participants so that each has an equal chance of being chosen (reduce sampling bias). This method is needed to ensure the accuracy of inferential statistical interpretation.
Random allocation	Method of assigning participants to groups using randomization (ie, flip a coin or random number generator) so each participant has an equal opportunity to be assigned to a given group. By using, greater confidence exists that the groups are equivalent at baseline. Also referred to as random assignment.
Independent variable	The variable the researcher is manipulating (active) or selecting (attribute) to determine the effect on the dependent variable
Dependent variable	The outcome variable of interest in a study; in research, the approach is taken that the independent variable influences the dependent variable.
Descriptive statistics	Statistics that summarize the characteristics of the data that include describing the center of the data (ie, mean and median) and variation (ie, standard deviation and range)
Inferential statistics	Statistics that are used to generalize (infer) the results of a study sample to the wider population
Type I error	The error committed when the data demonstrate a statistically significant result although no true difference or association exists in the population
Type II error	The error committed when the data do not demonstrate a statistically significance result when a true difference or association exists in the population
Alpha (α)	The probability, ideally established before inferential statistical analysis is conducted, that a type I statistical error will be permitted. Most frequently .05 is used.
Beta (β)	The probability, ideally established before inferential statistical analysis is conducted, that a type II statistical error will be permitted. Most frequently .20 is used.
Confidence interval	A range of values calculated from the sample data, which are likely to contain the value for the population to a given level of confidence. Most often 95% CI is used. The width of a confidence interval provides an indication of the precision of estimated population value, thereby assisting with determining clinical meaningfulness of statistical test results.

(continued on next page)

Table 1
(continued)

Term	Definition
Effect size	The observed or expected change or association between the 2 or more variables. Reporting standardized effect sizes (ie, *d* family or *r* family) can assist with determining clinical meaningfulness of statistical test results.
Measurement validity	The accuracy of a measure to quantify what it is designed to measure
Measurement error	The difference between the true value of a quality and what is measured
Measurement reliability	The quality of a measure to be consistent and free from measurement error
Minimal detectable difference	The minimal quantity of change that exceeds measurement error
Minimal important difference	Quantity of change that a patient perceives as worthwhile
Statistical power	The probability a statistical test will correctly identify a difference or association that truly exists (ie, not commit a type II statistical error)

combined, which has led to much of the P value interpretation confusion as well as many challenges to using P values to interpret the results of a research study.[1–3] Practitioners do not need a full understanding of the P value debate among statisticians. Rather, practitioners need to appreciate what a P value from an inferential statistic indicates and how to combine that information with other tools, such as confidence intervals and effect sizes, to evaluate the clinical meaningfulness of a research result.

In current practice, most research using inferential statistics with P values is done as a null hypothesis significance test (NHST). In conducting the inferential statistical test, a null hypothesis is created. A null hypothesis is frequently stated as there is no difference between groups (ie, the invention is not effective) or no relationship exists. It is critical to understand that the P value is a conditional probability; assuming a true null hypothesis, the P value provides the probability that the differences or relationships yielded by the sample data are attributable to sampling error. Although the P value was originally described as the magnitude of evidence against the null hypothesis (significance testing), in current practice the P value is often compared

Table 2
The average range of motion improvement for the 2 groups is identical; however, inspection of the individual responses demonstrates variability that is characterized by the standard deviation

Participant Number	Range of Motion Improvement (°)	
	Group 1	Group 2
1	8	5
2	10	18
3	13	2
4	10	15
5	9	10
Average ± SD	10 ± 1.9	10 ± 6.7

Table 3
Measurement scales and descriptive statistics

Measurement Scale	Definition	Examples	Measure of Center	Measure of Spread
Nominal	Unordered categories	Ethnicity, gender, injury status	Mode	Number of categories containing values
Ordinal	Ordered categories	Manual muscle test grades, reflex grades	Median	Interquartile range
Interval	Equal intervals between scores but no true zero	Temperature, time on a 12-h clock, GRE score	Mean[a]	Standard deviation[a]
Ratio	Equal intervals between scores and true zero	Body weight, blood pressure	Mean[a]	Standard deviation[a]

Abbreviation: GRE, graduate record examination.
[a] In cases of data not normally distributed or influential outliers, the median and interquartile range are more appropriate.

against a threshold point (α level) to make a binary decision to either reject or fail to reject the null hypothesis (NHST). When the computed P value is smaller than α, statistical significance, or rejection of the null hypothesis, is concluded. The α level is established by the researcher early in the research process; most often .05 is used, although there are circumstances where different α levels may be more appropriate.[4]

The process of making a yes-or-no decision regarding the null hypothesis by comparing the P value against α raises the possibility for making 2 kinds of errors. The first, referred to as a type I statistical error, is when the computed P value causes the researcher to reject a null hypothesis that was really true (ie, false positive). In this circumstance, the researcher is concluding that there is a difference or relationship when in reality there is not. The probability of making a type I error is related to the α level. The second type of statistical error, a type II error, occurs when the P value prompts a researcher to erroneously conclude there is no difference or relationship, thereby failing to reject a false null hypothesis (ie, false negative). The probability of making a type II statistical error is referred to as β. It is important to recognize that α and β do not indicate the likelihood that a single study has led to error but rather the likelihood over multiple replications of the research.[1]

To illustrate NHST and P value interpretation, consider a hypothetical study in which 2 different terminal-phase anterior cruciate ligament rehabilitation programs, conventional and accelerated, are compared for improving single-leg hop test limb symmetry index (LSI). In conducting the study, a random sample of 40 individuals who underwent anterior cruciate ligament reconstruction is randomly assigned to 1 of the 2 rehabilitation programs. After the 4-week terminal phase of rehabilitation, the participants' single-leg hop test LSI (uninjured/injured × 100) is determined. After the program, the LSI values are 87.3% ± 6.2% and 91.9% ± 6.5% for the conventional and accelerated groups, respectively. Based on the results of a statistical comparison between the groups ($t_{38} = 2.28$, $P = .028$), the researchers claim that the accelerated program is better than the conventional program because the computed P value was less than .05. The core of this interpretation is that the 4.6% LSI difference between the 2 rehabilitation groups exceeded what would be expected if no difference existed in the LSI improvements between the 2 groups.

Despite the common practice of NHST, as described previously, there are a few additional aspects that warrant consideration. First, despite the attractiveness of making a dichotomous decision (yes or no) regarding the null hypothesis, there is little logic in considering the findings of a study reporting a P value of .048 as evidence supporting an intervention whereas a P value of .052 leads to the conclusion that an intervention did not work because it was slightly larger than alpha, the statistically significant threshold. The P value is a function of several factors, including the sample size and the effect size. An effect size is the magnitude of the difference/change in relationship compared with the variability between the study participants (discussed later). Thus, in addition to considering the effect size, prudent practice also includes considering the P value in conjunction with the sample size.[5] Although a difference between groups may not reach statistical significance with a sample size of 10, the same difference becomes statistically significant with a sample size of 20 (**Table 4**).

STATISTICAL SIGNIFICANCE DOES NOT MEAN CLINICAL MEANINGFULNESS

Whereas statistical significance provides an indication of the role of chance on the outcome, clinical meaningfulness is the importance and relevance of the result to sports medicine practice. Demonstrating a significant improvement in an outcome measure (eg, pain) because of a clinical intervention (eg, rehabilitation) is worthwhile; however, if the change is very small and took 6 weeks of 3 rehabilitation sessions per week, it may be concluded that it does not have clinical meaningfulness. Thus, clinical meaningfulness is a subjective decision that weighs the risks and costs (eg, time and money) with the benefits yielded by a study that attained statistical significance. Additionally, when determining clinical meaningfulness, the reliability of the measurement tools and the types of participants used in the study also need to be considered. Although unreliable outcome measures decrease the likelihood of reaching statistical significance, if the changes deemed statistically significant do not exceed measurement error or what a patient perceives as beneficial, they may have little clinical meaningfulness. The MDD and MID are 2 tools to assist with this decision (discussed later). The characteristics of the study participants also influence the magnitude of change; smaller changes likely occur with interventions that use healthier participants versus more severely injured patients. Thus, in assessing clinical meaningfulness, a practitioner needs to evaluate the stated inclusion/exclusion criteria and the final characteristics of the participants, the relevance and reliability of the outcome measures, and the magnitude of the changes/differences revealed by the investigation.

Table 4
Effects of sample sizes on statistical significance and effect sizes

Sample Size	Mean Limb Symmetry Index Difference Between Groups (%)	t Statistic	P Value	Statistically Significant at .05?	Cohen's d Effect Size
10 per group	4.6	1.61	.116	No	.72
20 per group	4.6	2.28	.028	Yes	.72
30 per group	4.6	2.79	.008	Yes	.72

Unlike the P value, sample size does not influence the unstandardized (mean difference) or standardized (Cohen's d) effect sizes.

EFFECT SIZES AND CONFIDENCE INTERVALS AS MEASURES OF CLINICAL MEANINGFULNESS

Again, after a statistically significant result is determined, it is important to decide how clinically meaningful it is. One way to do this is using an effect size that estimates the magnitude of the changes or associations revealed by the statistical results. There are 2 main types of effect sizes: unstandardized and standardized. The unstandardized effect size is simply the mean difference of the outcome measures used within 1 study. Using the single-leg hop test, the unstandardized effect size is 4.6%, because this is the mean difference between the 2 groups (see **Table 4**). Although an unstandardized effect size can be interpreted directly, it cannot be compared across multiple studies. The standardized effect size is expressed on a unitless scale and, therefor,e can be used in a larger scope. The *d* family (difference between groups) and *r* family (association or relationship between variables) are 2 types of standardized effect sizes.

Although there are more than 70 different effect size indexes,[6] some of the most common in each of the families are focused on for this article. Cohen's *d* is the most common effect size in the *d* family. This effect size index is the mean difference between the 2 groups divided by the standard deviation (a standardizer). The standardizer is what places this type of effect size on a unitless scale. Researchers commonly use 3 categories of small (.2), medium (.5), and large (.8) when describing the effect size. A Cohen's *d* effect size of .72 (see **Table 4**) is computed using the single-leg hop test LSI data of 91.9% ± 6.5% (accelerated) and 87.3% ± 6.2% (conventional). The mean difference of 4.6 is divided by the pooled SD[7] of 6.38. Therefore, the individuals in the accelerated rehabilitation protocol had a higher LSI by .72 SDs than those in the conventional protocol. According to the categories presented by Cohen,[8] this represents a medium effect between the 2 rehabilitation programs. Cohen first suggested these classifications for psychology research where smaller effect sizes are more common than in sports medicine research. More recently, Rhea[9] suggested classifications for strength training research of less than .35 as trivial, .35 to .80 as small, .80 to 1.50 as moderate, and greater than 1.5 as large. Another common effect size in the *d* family is an odds ratio. If a clinician is interested in the association of the presence of reinjury with those individuals who completed the accelerated protocol compared with those in the conventional protocol, an odds ratio could be calculated. For example, with an odds ratio of .91, the individuals in each rehabilitation group have approximately equal odds of reinjury. An odds ratio of 1.00 is exactly equal odds.

When describing the practical importance using indexes from the *r* family, the more commonly seen options include a form of η^2 or a Pearson product moment correlation coefficient. η^2 is the proportion of the variation in the dependent variable explained by the independent variable. η^2 can be positively biased, especially for samples with fewer than 30 participants. An alternative is the partial eta squared (η^2_p), which accounts for the variation in the dependent variable and the associated independent variable of interest in isolation. The Pearson product moment correlation coefficient describes the relationship between 2 continuous variables. As an effect size, it defines the strength of the relationship. Bilateral strength imbalance (newton meter), specifically in the quadriceps, may be related with the LSI. Using a Pearson product moment correlation coefficient quantifies this relationship. For example, a finding of .89 suggests that there is a strong, positive correlation between these 2 measures.

Another way to determine clinical meaningfulness is with confidence intervals, which provide a range of possible values drawn from samples to estimate the population. With the example of the LSI scores after the 2 rehabilitation programs, the computed 95% CI suggests that the true population effect is between .51% and 8.67%. Confidence intervals can be considered at any level (eg, 90% or 99%), but the most commonly seen is 95%. This relates to the commonly seen use of $\alpha = .05$ as a determination of statistical significance. Similar to NHST, however, there is uncertainty (ie, role of chance = 5%) associated with this estimation. This implies that if samples were taken repeatedly, 95 times out of 100, the range would contain the population effect. The width of the confidence interval is determined based on the confidence a researcher must have in this decision-making process. Higher levels of confidence (99% CI vs 95% CI) produce wider confidence intervals. In addition to the level of confidence, sample size and the variability in the data also have an impact on the width of the confidence interval. As discussed previously, the P value only indicates statistical significance. In contrast, confidence interval can assess both statistical and clinical significance. If a 95% CI for the mean difference contains zero, there is no difference between the 2 groups. Contrary, if the 95% CI does not contain zero, there is a statistically significant difference. **Table 5** provides 3 examples of research questions, the statistical techniques best suited for answering the questions, and the reporting of statistical findings, including effect sizes, and confidence intervals.

UNDERSTANDING MINIMAL DETECTABLE DIFFERENCE AND MINIMAL IMPORTANT DIFFERENCE

Although understanding reliability, the extent to which a measure is free of error, may seem simplistic, it is a challenging concept to decipher. There are 2 types of errors: systematic and random error. These added together are the total measurement error associated with a measure. Systematic errors could occur due to factors, such as learning effects or participant fatigue across multiple trials, whereas random errors take place due to biological, mechanical, or research protocol changes. There are 3 frequently used statistical methods to report reliability: relative reliability (ie, test-retest correlation), systematic bias (ie, change in mean), and absolute reliability (ie, repeated measurement variability).[10,11] Relative reliability is the consistency of an individual's position within a group over several measurements. The intraclass correlation coefficient is commonly seen within sports medicine literature as a measure of relative reliability (ranging from 0 to 1, with 1 perfect relative reliability). Systematic bias can be reported using a paired t test (2 measurements) or a repeated measures analysis of variance (3 or more measurements). Although relative reliability and systematic bias are important, absolute reliability may have more clinical relevance. Absolute reliability indicates variability in repeated measurements for an individual. Standard error of measurement (SEM) is 1 method of determining absolute reliability. The SEM is typically seen when the intraclass correlation coefficient is presented. In a similar manner, the MDD also provides measurement error boundaries; however, it is more conservative (wider error boundaries) than the SEM. Any change that occurs outside the MDD boundaries can be considered more appropriately as real change. The MID is the level of change, beyond the MDD, that a patient perceives to be meaningful and at which the patient would repeat the treatment again.[12] Two approaches are used to determine the MID, anchor based (an external criterion is used to determine if a meaningful change has occurred or not) and distribution based (statistical significant change, precision of the measurement, or variability in the scores). The second approach is more statistical in nature and does not account for patient preference as much as the anchor-based methods. The anchor-based methods, however, lack the generalizability of the distribution-based approach. There is little agreement in

Table 5

Statistical approaches frequently seen in literature with the common assumptions, typical reporting of statistical findings, and clinical interpretation to assist a practitioner reading a research article

Research Question	Analytical Technique	Common Assumptions	Statistical Findings	Clinical Interpretation
Is there an association between injury location (knee or hip) and abnormal LSI (asymmetry $\geq 15\%$ or asymmetry $<15\%$)?	Chi-square test of association	Observations are independent; expected frequency is at least 5 per cell	$\chi^2_1 = 0.400$, $P = .527$, $R = 0.10$, 95% CI (-0.208, 0.390)	There is no association between the location of injury and abnormal LSI results.
Is there a difference in LSI depending on type of sport (soccer, basketball, or football)?	One-way ANOVA with Tukey post hoc testing	Observations are independent; homogeneity of variance; populations follow a normal distribution	$F_{2,37} = 1.674$, $P = .015$, 95% CI (87.311, 91.870), $\eta^2_p = 0.20$; football to basketball: $P = .035$	There is a difference in LSI based on the type of sport, specifically between football and basketball athletes.
Do gender, age, and LSI predict time to RTP after a quadriceps strain?	Multiple linear regression	Observations are independent; homogeneity of variance; normal distribution; linearity; noncollinearity;	$F_{3,36} = 2.990$, $P = .044$, $R^2 = 0.20$; LSI: $t = 2.241$, $P = .031$, 95% CI: (0.011, 0.0229)	The overall model (gender, age, and LSI) can predict days until RTP in those athletes with a quadriceps strain; specifically, LSI is statistically significant.

When statistical results are reported, it is customary to report the value of the test statistic (ie, F, t, and χ^2) and the degrees of freedom as a subscript. Effect sizes (ie, d, R, η^2_p, and R^2), and confidence intervals (upper and lower boundaries separated by a comma) appear after the P values.

Abbreviations: ANOVA, analysis of variance; R^2, coefficient of determination; RTP, return to play.

literature on which approach is superior.[13–16] A practical example of using the MDD and MID for interpreting a patients' change in shoulder pain has recently been provided.[17]

INTERPRETING STUDIES THAT DO NOT REACH STATISTICAL SIGNIFICANCE

Currently, there exists a publication bias, with largely only articles yielding statistically significant positive results published.[18–20] The bias is likely a combination of researchers hesitant to submit research with nonsignificant results and journal editorial boards tending to accept articles only with statistically significant results. Regardless of the source, the outcome presents a challenge when conducting systematic reviews and meta-analyses because only studies with statistical significance, and likely large effect sizes, are available for consideration. For example, in the context of sports medicine research examining various interventions for injury prevention and recovery, this may lead to an overestimation of the benefits various interventions may have on preventing injury and improving patient function. Thus, it is important that high-quality studies with nonsignificant findings be published; the challenge is how to evaluate whether such studies meet the bar for high quality.

Statistical power is the probability of attaining statistical significance ($P<\alpha$) and not committing a type II statistical error. In other words, statistical power is the likelihood of rejecting a false null hypothesis and making an appropriate statistical decision. Statistical power is influenced by the α level, sample size, and magnitude of the treatment effect relative to the variation in how the participants responded to the treatments (ie, effect size). As discussed previously, an α level of .05 is standard practice. In cases of intervention studies, the magnitude of the treatment effect and response variation is largely a function of the intervention parameters selected, such as dosage (eg, how many rehabilitation sessions per week), as well as the participant inclusion and exclusion criteria (eg, severity and variability in pathology). It is easier to achieve statistical significance when there are large effects and little variation in the response to the treatment. Sample size is the power parameter that often receives the most attention during the study planning process. Prudent practice is to conduct an a priori power analysis to estimate how many participants are needed to reach statistical significance given chosen values for the α level, statistical power (.80 is most common), and the anticipated effect size. Preferably, the anticipated effect size should be based on what is considered a clinically relevant change. Using the MDD or MID can help with selecting an effect size that is clinically relevant. Previous literature and pilot studies can also provide guidance regarding the potential potency of an intervention. Although an a priori power analysis can be conducted by using the standard interpretation conventions, described previously (eg, Cohen's d classifications), the authors suggest avoiding this approach in isolation because it does not consider the clinical relevance of the change.

Readers of research should look for evidence of an a priori power analysis, particularly in studies reporting nonsignificant results. In the circumstance of nonstatistically significant results, evaluation needs to occur to determine which of the following is more tenable: (1) Is there truly no difference in the effectiveness of the treatment interventions? or (2) Is there a possibility that type II statistical error has occurred? Along with examining other elements of the research design and execution, the details of an a priori power analysis can help with this evaluation. If an a priori power analysis is not included or if insufficient detail regarding the statistical power analysis is provided, determining which of the 2 scenarios, discussed previously, is more likely cannot occur. **Box 1** contains some guidance for evaluating an a priori analysis.

Box 1
Some considerations for evaluating an a priori statistical power analysis

Were the chosen alpha and power levels appropriate?

Is there sufficient detail regarding the source of the difference and variance estimates to evaluate? If yes:
  Do the difference/variance (ie, effect size) have clinical relevance?
  If previous research/pilot studies were used to assist, was the population similar to the current study?
  Was there some buffer to account for sampling fluctuation included?

In cases of an intervention study failing to reach statistical significance, assuming the research was well designed and executed, answering "yes" to each of the questions suggests there being truly no effect or a smaller than anticipated effect.

Finally, even with an optimally conducted a priori power analysis to establish sample size prior to commencing the research, it is still possible that non–statistically significant results could be due to a type II statistical error. Again, research relies on sampling from populations and, therefore, the study sample may demonstrate higher variability than the power analysis estimate or illicit less response to the intervention than the population. Thus, similar to needing study replication when statistically significant results occur to provide more evidence against a possible type 1 error, well-conducted investigations with solid rationale that fail to reach statistical significance may also warrant independent replication to rule out a possible type II error.

SUMMARY

Few practitioners enter sports medicine with a desire to develop an extensive understanding of statistics; however, as part of the EBP movement, practitioners must have some competency in understanding research. Interpreting the statistical analysis and results is an important component of that competency. This article provides some of the minimal statistical essentials sports medicine practitioners can use to facilitate understanding of research reports. Statistical significance, as reflected by a P value associated with a statistical test, indicates the influence of chance on the outcome, whereas clinical meaningfulness reflects the degree to which the study results reported are relevant to sports medicine practice. When statistically significant differences are revealed, confidence intervals and effect sizes can be used to enhance the practical interpretation of the research results. Absolute reliability characteristics, such as the MDD, determine the extent of error around a measurement and, when coupled with an appropriate MID estimate, can assist in triangulating clinically meaningful changes in patients undergoing treatment. In the circumstance of nonstatistically significant results, evaluation needs to occur to determine if the study had adequate statistical power prior to concluding the data are indicating that no difference or association exists in the population. Better understanding of these research and statistical concepts will improve EBP and, therefore, patient care.

REFERENCES

1. Goodman S. Toward evidenced-based medical statistics. 1: the P value fallacy. Ann Intern Med 1999;130:995–1004.
2. Kline R. Beyond significance testing: statistical reform in the behaviorial sciences. 2nd edition. Washington, DC: American Psychological Association; 2013.

3. Blume J, Peipert J. What your statistician never told you about P-values. J Am Assoc Gynecol Laparosc 2003;10(4):439–44.

4. Huck S. Reading statistics and research. Boston: Pearson Education, Inc; 2012.

5. Riemann BL, Lininger M. Statistical primer for athletic trainers: the difference between statistical and clinical meaningfulness. J Athl Train 2015;50(12):1223–5.

6. Kirk ER. The importance of effect magnitude. In: Davis S, editor. Handbook of research methods in experimental psychology. Oxford (United Kingdom): Blackwell; 2003. p. 83–105.

7. Lininger M, Riemann BL. Statistical primer for athletic trainers: using confidence intervals and effect sizes to evaluate clinical meaningfulness. J Athl Train 2016; 51(12):1045–8.

8. Cohen J. Statistical power analysis for the behavioral sciences. 2nd edition. Hillsdale (NJ): Lawrence Erlbaum Associations, Publishers; 1988.

9. Rhea MR. Determining the magnitude of treatment effects in strength training research through the use of the effect size. J Strength Cond Res 2004;18(4): 918–20.

10. Atkinson G, Nevill AM. Statistical methods for assessing measurement error (reliability) in variables relevant to sports medicine. Sports Med 1998;26(4):217–38.

11. Hopkins WG, Hawley JA, Burke LM. Design and analysis of research on sport performance enhancement. Med Sci Sports Exerc 1999;31(3):472–85.

12. Copay AG, Subach BR, Glassman SD, et al. Understanding the minimum clinically important difference: a review of concepts and methods. Spine J 2007; 7(5):541–6.

13. Crosby RD, Kolotkin RL, Williams GR. Defining clinically meaningful change in health-related quality of life. J Clin Epidemiol 2003;56(5):395–407.

14. de Vet HC, Terluin B, Knol DL, et al. Three ways to quantify uncertainty in individually applied "minimally important change" values. J Clin Epidemiol 2010;63(1): 37–45.

15. King MT. A point of minimal important difference (MID): a critique of terminology and methods. Expert Rev Pharmacoecon Outcomes Res 2011;11(2):171–84.

16. Sloan JA. Assessing the minimally clinically significant difference: scientific considerations, challenges and solutions. COPD 2005;2(1):57–62.

17. Riemann B, Lininger M. Statistical primer for athletic trainers: the essentials of understanding measures of reliability and minimal important change. J Athl Train 2018;53(1):98–103.

18. Hopewell S, Loudon K, Clarke MJ, et al. Publication bias in clinical trials due to statistical significance or direction of trial results. Cochrane Database Syst Rev 2009;(1). MR000006.

19. Joober R, Schmitz N, Annable L, et al. Publication bias: what are the challenges and can they be overcome? J Psychiatry Neurosci 2012;37(3):149–52.

20. Torgerson C. Publication bias: the Achilles' heel of systematic reviews? Br J Educ Stud 2006;54(1):89–102.

Fundamentals of Sports Analytics

Erin B. Wasserman, PhD[a],*, Mackenzie M. Herzog, MPH[b,c],
Christy L. Collins, PhD[a], Sarah N. Morris, PhD[a], Stephen W. Marshall, PhD[d]

KEYWORDS

- Epidemiology • Study design • Analytics • Sports performance • Injury occurrence

KEY POINTS

- There are a variety of research study designs that can be used to identify risk factors for injury, including cohort, case control, and case series.
- Each has advantages and disadvantages and their use should be determined by the data available and the research question at hand.
- Sports injury surveillance systems are useful for collecting injury incidence data but have unique limitations.
- Common analytical measures used in sports injury research include injury rate, injury risk and odds, incidence rate ratio, and risk difference and can be calculated based on the study design and research question.
- There has been increased emphasis on using technology to measure athletic performance, but much is still unknown about best practices with these data.

INTRODUCTION

Analytics, in some form or another, have always been a part of sports. Basic statistics, such as the score of the game, or the number of receptions or hits, provide the basis for athletic competition. Recently, however, the importance of statistics and analytics in sports has increased, with emphasis on measures that improve the likelihood of winning or may provide an "edge" over the competition who has not yet discovered the value of these measures. These analytics include measures of sport aptitude

Disclosure Statement: No conflicts of interest to disclose.
[a] Datalys Center for Sports Injury Research and Prevention, Inc, 401 West Michigan Street, Suite 500, Indianapolis, IN 46202, USA; [b] Department of Epidemiology, The University of North Carolina at Chapel Hill, Suite 500, Bank of America Building 7505, Chapel Hill, NC 27599, USA; [c] Real-World Evidence, IQVIA, Research Triangle Park, 4820 Emperor Boulevard, Durham, NC 27703, USA; [d] Department of Epidemiology, The University of North Carolina at Chapel Hill, Injury Prevention Research Center, Suite 500, Bank of America Building 7505, Chapel Hill, NC 27599, USA
* Corresponding author.
E-mail address: ewasserman@datalyscenter.org

(eg, strikeouts in baseball, free-throw percentage in basketball), physical location (eg, pitch location in baseball, distance run in basketball), economic value, and, most relevant to medicine, injury incidence and metrics of physical performance.

Just as measures of sport aptitude have been used in the sports setting to increase win probability, there is increasing recognition that understanding injury occurrence and identifying factors that can prevent injury can provide a team with an advantage on the field or court via implementation of data-driven injury prevention strategies. Additionally, recent advances in technology have led to an improved understanding of physical ability, functional movement, training load, and fatigue. Understanding an athlete's workload can lead to improved training that maximizes athletic performance and minimizes fatigue and injury.

The emphasis of this review is to describe measures of sports injury and fundamentals of sports injury research with a brief overview of some of the emerging measures of sports performance. First, we describe research study designs that can be used to identify risk factors for injury. Second, we discuss an important source of injury incidence data: surveillance programs. Third, we describe common measures of injury risk and association. Finally, we describe measures of physical performance and training and considerations for using these measures. This review provides sports medicine clinicians with an understanding of current research measures and considerations for designing sports injury research studies.

SPORTS INJURY RESEARCH STUDY DESIGNS

The goal of research is to answer a question about a broader population using a sample of data. Here, the population is the entire group that we want to study (eg, all adolescent boys' basketball players in the United States), and the study sample is a subset (eg, a sample of United States high school boys' basketball teams) that we actually examine to make an inference about the population of interest. Our ability to answer research questions depends on the strength of the study design, including the overall framework used, the validity of the data collected, and the rigor of the analysis and interpretation.

Evidence can be generated from both experimental and observational study designs. Experimental studies, such as randomized controlled trials, are largely considered the gold standard for evidence generation owing to the validity afforded by randomization, that is, the ability to balance participant characteristics that may affect the outcome of interest ("confounders") between groups, control treatment, or exposure delivery, and isolate treatment effects among specific populations of interest.[1–3] However, randomized controlled trials and other experimental study designs also have limitations, including high costs and time required for study completion, potential lack of real-world applicability and generalizability, a need for equipoise, and an exposure that can be ethically randomized.[1–3] Owing to these caveats, many research questions cannot be answered using experimental study designs.

Observational studies can also generate high-quality evidence when rigorous research methods are used. These studies typically fall within 3 broad study designs: cohort, case control, and case series studies (**Table 1**).[1,3] Here we provide a high-level overview of the fundamental concepts underpinning these study designs. These study designs can be used with data stemming from a variety of sources, including surveillance data, electronic medical records, administrative claims or billing information, or data specifically collected for research purposes, and the source of the data and study design are not inherently linked together, but rather separate concepts.

Cohort Studies

The basis of a cohort study involves following a group of individuals who arise from the population we want to study, some of whom are exposed to an intervention, characteristic, or experience and some of whom are unexposed. Exposure has been assigned by some nonrandom process, such as some individual choosing to wear a personal protective equipment item (eg, mouthguard), whereas others choose not to wear the item. These individuals are followed forward in time to observe an outcome of interest.[1–3] A cohort study can be initiated either prospectively or retrospectively. In a prospective study, subjects are enrolled and then followed forward in time. In a retrospective cohort study, the sample is still selected based on exposure, but the exposures are identified after the outcome event occurs, even though the exposure was recorded before the event occurring. In essence, all cohorts are prospective in time. Thus, the term "historical" cohort study is sometimes used instead of "retrospective."

In sports studies, the exposure could be anything from an athlete characteristic (eg, age, body mass index, gender, alignment, anatomic structure), to a playing condition (eg, field type, footwear, weather, sport schedule), to an intervention intended to reduce injury risk (eg, warm-up program, bracing, taping, safety equipment, rule changes), or even prior injury history or prior treatment for injury. The outcome is typically an injury, reinjury, or other adverse player health event, although the outcome could also be time lost from participation, return to sport, performance level, medical disqualification from sport, or the need for surgical intervention or other treatment.

The ultimate purpose of a cohort study is to determine whether the exposure of interest is associated with outcome occurrence.[2,3] As such, all members of the cohort must be outcome negative (free of the outcome) at the start of the follow-up period, so that temporality between the exposure and outcome occurrence is clearly defined.[1,3]

Table 1
Comparison of study design features for cohort, case control, and case series studies

Cohort	Case Control	Case Series
Anchored in time based on exposure	Anchored in time based on outcome	Descriptive based on outcome positive status
Must include both an exposed and unexposed group at the start of follow-up	Must include both an outcome positive and outcome negative group at the start of the study	Only includes an outcome positive group
Participants followed forward in time from exposure of interest to outcome	Exposure determined retrospectively after identification of outcome or no outcome	Exposures described after outcome positive group is identified
Both exposed and unexposed must be at risk for the outcome for duration of follow-up	Both exposed and unexposed must be at risk for the outcome for duration of follow-up	Only includes an outcome positive group—timing of exposure and outcome described
Cohort members must be outcome negative at the start of follow-up	Study participants must be outcome negative at the time of exposure	Study participants must be outcome positive
Study can be initiated either prospectively or retrospectively	Study can be initiated either prospectively or retrospectively	Study can be initiated either prospectively or retrospectively

Another important feature of the cohort study is "exchangeability" of the exposed and unexposed groups; the unexposed group should be similar to the exposed in all other aspects other than exposure.[3] For example, suppose we wish to assess the effect of helmets on concussion incidence. The exposed group includes football players who wear helmets, whereas the unexposed group includes tennis players who do not wear helmets. In this scenario, it would be difficult to determine whether a difference in concussion incidence was due to helmet use or due to the background difference in concussion incidence and many other characteristics that differ between football and tennis players and their respective sports.

In observational research studies, where participants are identified from a non-randomized, real-world setting, it is often difficult to ensure that the exposed and unexposed groups are truly exchangeable.[2,3] Analytical and design methods can be used to account for potential confounders if these characteristics are enumerated and quantified. In-depth discussion of methods for adjusting for confounders is outside the scope of this review paper, but these techniques include restriction, stratification, matching, standardization, or analytical adjustment. Analytical adjustment using a statistical model is a common strategy that can be implemented if these factors are carefully considered before study initiation and the data are available.[1,3]

Case Control Studies

Similar to the cohort study, the goal of a case control study is also to determine whether the exposure of interest is associated with outcome occurrence. Case control studies, however, identify participants based on the outcome rather than the exposure, comparing individuals who are outcome positive to those who are outcome negative.[1,3] Case control studies are efficient study designs for rare events owing to the selection of cases driving the study sample. As in the cohort study, the study group for a case control study must also arise from the total population of interest.[1,3] In other words, every case control study takes place within the context of (or is "nested" in) a hypothetical cohort. After the study sample is identified, the investigator compares the prevalence of the exposure before the index date for the outcome positive and outcome negative groups.[1,3] For example, at the end of a basketball season, we may select basketball players from 1 team who sustained an ankle sprain compared with players on that team who did not sustain an ankle sprain, and then look backward in time to determine how many in each group participated in an injury prevention program during preseason.[4]

Logically, the key considerations for a cohort study that are listed, including being outcome negative at the time of exposure, exchangeability between the 2 groups (here, the outcome positive and outcome negative groups), and adjustment for confounders, also apply to case control studies. However, there are several additional considerations for case control studies, including the conscious selection of a strategy for selection of controls that is appropriate for the research question of interest.[1,3]

Controls must always arise from the source population of interest, and they can be selected using one of 3 different methods.

First, among the full study cohort (eg, all basketball players participating at the start of the season) that includes all the exposed and unexposed among the study sample, controls can be sampled from the total cohort, which would include outcome positive individuals.[1,3] This type of sampling is preferred because it represents the full cohort; however, it is typically only used if collection of data is time consuming or expensive, limiting the opportunity to perform an analysis of the full cohort. This control selection strategy is often referred to as "case cohort" sampling.

Second, control sampling can be performed from a group of outcome negative individuals who meet exchangeability criteria for the outcome positive individuals (eg, basketball players who did not sustain an ankle sprain by the end of the season).[1,3]

Third, control sampling can be performed in a prospective and dynamic fashion, such that among a group of individuals followed over time, and, when a case is identified, a control is also selected from the group at the same point in time (eg, when an ankle sprain occurs, select another basketball player playing in the same game who has not sustained ankle sprain).[1,3] With this method of sampling, it is possible that some individuals selected as controls may later become cases.[1,3] This control selection strategy is often referred to as "risk set" or "cohort nested" sampling and is conceptually closely linked to the prospective cohort study in which most of noncases are "missing by design."[4]

Regardless of how controls are sampled for a case control study, it is imperative that they be selected without respect to the exposure status (eg, controls should be taken without considering whether they participated in the prevention program during preseason). Failure to adhere to this requirement results in a biased estimate of the effect of the exposure on the outcome of interest.[1,3]

Case Series

The defining feature that differentiates a case series study from a cohort study is the lack of an outcome negative group.[5] In a case series, a group of individuals who are all outcome positive is analyzed.[5] For example, a group of injured athletes may be studied to determine the average time to return to play after the injury of interest, or a group of individuals who underwent a surgical procedure may be assessed to determine the proportion who need a revision procedure. These studies are valuable for describing the characteristics or outcomes of a group; however, it is important to note that the relationship between the characteristic, outcome, or other variable of interest and the experience that determined case series membership, cannot be assessed.[5] For example, if we study a series of soccer players who sustained an anterior cruciate ligament rupture and note that 80% of these players were participating on field turf at the time of injury, this does not suggest that field turf increases likelihood of anterior cruciate ligament rupture. To answer that question, we would need to also understand either the distribution of field turf participation for all soccer players or for a sample of uninjured soccer players. Nevertheless, this type of descriptive study is often the first step in hypothesis generation that can motivate performing a future in-depth investigation into an association.

SPORTS INJURY SURVEILLANCE

As noted, the data for all these study designs can be derived from a variety of sources. One common source of these data are sports injury surveillance systems. Sports injury surveillance systems can examine trends in sports injuries over time and measure the impact of interventions aimed to reduce sports injuries. Injury surveillance is the "ongoing and systematic collection" of injury data.[6,7] Surveillance systems exist in a variety of settings to collect a multitude of data, including hospital admissions and mortality, and many sports injury surveillance systems have been established at the high school,[8–10] collegiate,[11] and professional[12–14] levels. In addition to descriptive data, surveillance systems can be used as the source of cases and controls in case control studies. Surveillance systems can also be used for cohort studies, either retrospective in nature using data already collected, or they can be used to track outcomes among subjects enrolled prospectively into a study.

Injury surveillance is most commonly used for assessing the incidence of various conditions in different sports settings and addressing trends over time. These assessments can be used to demonstrate the need for research on a particular injury type, sport, or play. Among clinicians, measurements of injury incidence are used to justify their roles and help to determine resource allocation of clinical services and equipment.[15] These assessments are also used to justify the implementation of an intervention or rule change by governing bodies.[11] Once the intervention or rule change is implemented, injury surveillance can determine the impact of the intervention on injury occurrence by continuously monitoring injury rates over time or retrospectively assessing injury rates preimplementation and postimplementation.[16]

Although there are many uses and strengths of sports injury surveillance, there are also limitations and considerations for using surveillance data to answer sports injury research questions (**Table 2**). Sports injury surveillance is instrumental in establishing the "who, what, when, and where" of sports injuries. However, to capture large volumes of data, data collection processes are often streamlined and focus on breadth rather than depth. Therefore, etiology, especially at the individual level, is difficult to establish. Unlike a traditional prospective cohort study, individuals do not typically have baseline measurements and may not be followed over time. Rather, data are collected at a population level and focus on the injuries and the circumstances surrounding the injuries, often with only group-level measurements of time at risk.

Some existing sports injury surveillance systems have data available for release to external researchers for peer-reviewed publications. These include the Consumer Product Safety Commission's National Electronic Injury Surveillance System,[17] the NCAA Injury Surveillance Program,[11] and the National Athletic Treatment, Injury and Outcomes Network.[10] Whether using an existing sports injury surveillance system to answer a new research question or implementing your own sports injury surveillance system, it is important to consider a number of factors that influence the way data from these systems are interpreted. These include the following factors.

- *Definition of the injury*: How is an "injury" defined? Must the injury be related to a sports activity? Are both time loss and non–time loss injuries included? Are multiple injuries from the same injury event included? Some examples of injury definitions are included in **Table 3**.

Table 2
Strengths and limitations of sports injury surveillance

Strengths	Limitations
Establishes extent of the injury problem, including incidence and severity[16]	Many etiologic factors not captured, especially at the individual level
Consistent data collection over time to capture trends	Difficult to adapt data collection for changes in clinical practice or sport play without affecting time trends
Intervention effectiveness can be determined	Data collection often not specific to particular injuries, sports, or plays (breadth prioritized over depth)
Data can be captured using means integrated with clinical documentation (easy data collection)	Research definitions for variables not always used; consistency of data collection across sites unknown
Population-level estimates derived	Individuals usually not followed longitudinally; traditional cohort study analyses may be inappropriate

Table 3
Possible definitions of "injury" in sports injury surveillance systems

Full Definition	Short Definition
Any injury or physical complaint sustained by a player that affects or limits participation in any aspect of sport-related activity[14]	Impeded participation
An injury that occurred as a result of participation in an organized practice or competition, required attention from an AT or physician, and resulted in restriction of the student–athlete's participation for ≥1 d beyond the day of injury[8,11]	Medically attended, ≥1 d time lost
Any injury that was evaluated or treated (or both) by an AT or physician, regardless of time lost[11]	All medically attended
Any injury that prevents a player from taking a full part in all training and competition play activities typically planned for that day for a period of >24 h from midnight at the end of the day the injury was sustained[18]	Medically attended, >1 d time lost
All injuries resulting in a player missing ≥1 competitive competition[18]	Prevented participation in a competition
Any physical or medical condition that causes a player to miss a competition in the regular season or finals (playoffs)[12]	Prevented participation in a competition (regular/postseason)

Abbreviation: AT, athletic trainer.

- *Data source*: Are the data collected from a clinical system (eg, integration with an electronic medical record) or from a separate system designed for research purposes? Is the data collector a clinician (eg, athletic trainer) or someone trained to perform research studies? How are the data collectors trained? What is the likelihood of missing data and how are these data handled?
- *Population and sample*: Is this a sample or a census? If a sample of the population is taken, how was this sample taken; was it a simple random sample (teams/schools are selected using a some form of random process and have a predetermined fixed probability of being selected), a stratified random sample (same as a simple random sample, except the probability of selection varies based on some larger group of which they are a part; eg, geographic region, size, league), or a convenience sample (any team/school that volunteers to participate is included)?
- *Denominator*: How is time at risk captured? Is it at the individual level or the population level? Is it by hours or minutes of play or unit-based (eg, athlete–exposure)?

There is no right or wrong answer for many of these questions, but each has implications for how data should be analyzed and interpreted.

COMMON MEASURES OF INJURY OCCURRENCE AND ASSOCIATION WITH RISK
Injury Rate

The most frequently used metric of injury occurrence in sports injury research is a rate, which describes the number of injuries divided by the total time that the study population was at risk for injury.[19] An athlete–exposure (AE) denominator is one of the most commonly used measures of time at risk in the literature, with this metric representing one athlete participating in one athletic event, such as a practice, game, or conditioning session.[19,20]

$$Rate = \frac{\sum injuries}{\sum AEs}$$

The resulting interpretation of the incidence rate is, "X number of injuries are expected to occur for every X number of AEs."

Aside from an AE denominator, there are multiple other metrics that can be used to describe the time that athletes are at risk for injury, which are summarized in **Table 4**. The choice of a denominator depends on the research question of interest and the preferred method of describing and communicating injury occurrence, as well as availability of data. In many cases, the most granular information on participation is preferred (eg, player–minute of participation) because these data provide the most accurate description of time at risk; however, these data are rarely available across all settings (eg, both practices and games). Subsequently, the strengths and limitations of the denominator of choice should always be considered and summarized when presenting results.

The primary benefit of calculating an injury rate versus another injury occurrence metric is the ability to account for varying time at risk for injury between players, teams, or other groups.[19] For example, when comparing game injuries among first string versus second string players, second string players are likely to have a lower injury risk per game than first string players because they play for less time in each game. Accounting for the difference in minutes played between first and second string players by calculating a rate per player–minute creates more comparable groups in terms of time at risk when assessing injury occurrence. An additional benefit of the rate metric is the ability to allow for inclusion of all injuries, including multiple injuries to the same athlete, in the numerator.[19] Athletes reenter the pool of time at risk as soon as they are once again eligible to sustain an injury.

With the ability to measure all injuries, including multiple injuries to the same athlete, this brings up additional considerations for defining recurrent injuries,

Table 4
Rate denominators for sports injury studies

Denominator	Assumptions
Team—season	Across all teams participating, the baseline risk for injury is the same across a season; Can include injuries that occur in any setting (eg, practices, games, training) in the numerator
Team—games	Across all teams participating, the baseline risk for injury is the same across a game; should only include injuries that occur in a game in the numerator
Player—season	Across all players participating, the baseline risk for injury is the same across a season; can include injuries that occur in any setting (eg, practices, games, training) in the numerator
Player—games	Across all players participating, the baseline risk for injury is the same across a game; should only include injuries that occur in a game in the numerator
Player—minutes or player—plays	Assumes players are only at risk for injury while they are actively participating; should only include injuries that occur while participation is measured
Athlete—exposure (1 athlete participating in 1 athletic practice, competition, or training session)	Similar to player—games, assumes the baseline risk for injury is the same across each athletic session; can include injuries that occur in any setting (eg, practices, games, training) in the numerator

new/subsequent injuries, or exacerbations of a previous injury. Generally, a subsequent injury is any injury that occurs after a first injury, irrespective of whether it is related to earlier injury occurrences. A recurrent injury is another injury of the same type at the same location, and an exacerbation is a reinjury before resolution of the prior injury.[21,22] Finch and Cook's[21] subsequent injury categorization model had become a standard for use in classifying these injuries, providing even more detailed definitions of subsequent injuries, broken down into 10 categories. In many cases, however, the information needed for using the subsequent injury categorization model is not available, and researchers must rely on the clinical judgment of data collectors.

Injury Risk and Odds

Although injury rates are most commonly used to describe and compare injury occurrence, injury risk provides a metric that is more easily interpreted and communicated to stakeholders who are not scientists or data analysts (eg, players, coaches, administrators, general public).[19] Injury risk is the average probability across all athletes that an athlete will sustain an injury over a specific time period of participation.[20] In sports, injury risk is most frequently used to describe the number of athletes who sustain at least one injury over the course of a season of participation:

$$\text{Injury Risk for a Season} = \frac{\text{Number of injured athletes in a season}}{\text{Number of athletes at risk of being injured in a season}}$$

This metric can also be used to describe the risk of injury in any given game, assuming that all athletes on the team are at risk for injury for the entire game, regardless of their actual participation time. Injury risk is a more intuitive concept to grasp than injury rate because it is bounded by 0 and 1 and can be expressed as a percentage[19]; however, the calculation of risk also requires that the athlete is both observed for the full time period and at risk for injury during the full time period.[1,3] Additionally, multiple injuries to the same athlete during the same risk period (eg, 1 season or 1 game) are not included in the numerator, because the numerator counts injured athletes (not injuries). Differences in playing time or, in the case of risk across a season, number of events in which the athlete participated, are also not accounted for in the denominator used in injury risk. In addition, calculation of risk assumes that all athletes analyzed have a comparable baseline risk for injury over the time period of interest. This assumption should be carefully considered when using risk metrics, because the validity of the assumption may be questioned for certain comparisons, such as first string versus second string players. Nevertheless, calculating percentages of athletes who sustain an injury over a sports season is important for understanding and comparing the burden of sports injuries.

Similarly, the odds of injury, which is a function of risk, is another metric that can be used to describe injury occurrence.

$$\text{Injury odds for a season} = \frac{\text{Risk}}{(1 - \text{Risk})}$$

$$= \frac{\dfrac{\text{Number of injured athletes in a season}}{\text{Number of athletes at risk of being injured in a season}}}{\left(1 - \dfrac{\text{Number of injured athletes in a season}}{\text{Number of athletes at risk of being injured in a season}}\right)}$$

Similar to risk, calculating odds requires that the athlete is both observed for the full time period and at risk for injury during the full time period; however, odds are bounded by 0 and ∞, rather than 0 and 1.[1,3] Calculation of risk is typically preferred over odds, because risk is more intuitive and odds tend to be more extreme than risk.[3]

Measures of Association

Measures of association can be used to compare injury rates, risks, and odds between 2 groups of interest, such as the exposed and unexposed in cohort studies or the cases and controls in case control studies. These measures are used to identify factors associated with increased or decreased injury incidence. A ratio measure is calculated by taking the measure of occurrence in the exposed or cases and dividing by the measure of occurrence in the unexposed or controls. As an example calculation, an incidence rate ratio (IRR) is calculated as follows.

$$IRR = \frac{Rate_{exposed}}{Rate_{unexposed}} = \frac{\dfrac{\sum injuries}{\sum AEs}\ exposed}{\dfrac{\sum injuries}{\sum AEs}\ Unexposed}$$

For ratio measures, if no association exists between the exposure and the outcome, the resulting point estimate will be approximately 1, or a null association.[1,3] The point estimate from a ratio measure is interpreted as, "the risk/rate/odds of injury among the exposed/cases is x times the risk/rate/odds of injury among the unexposed/controls."

Comparable ratio measures can be computed for odds and risk. Notably, the odds ratio is the only measure of association that can be calculated directly from case control studies, because the calculation of a rate ratio or risk ratio requires information about the denominator or total study population at risk.[1] In a case control study, a sample of controls is selected from the study population at risk instead. However, depending on the sampling strategy used for control selection, the odds ratio may approximate the risk or rate ratio. A case control study that uses case cohort sampling estimates a risk ratio, whereas case control study that uses risk set sampling estimates a rate ratio.

Ratios provide relative measures of association between 2 groups. Difference measures, on the other hand, provide absolute measures of association. A rate or risk difference can be calculated by taking the rate or risk in the exposed and subtracting the rate or risk in the unexposed. As an example calculation, a risk difference (RD) is calculated as follows.

$$RD = Risk_{exposed} - Risk_{unexposed}$$
$$= \frac{Number\ of\ injured\ athletes\ in\ a\ season}{Number\ of\ athletes\ at\ risk\ of\ being\ injured\ in\ a\ season}_{exposed}$$
$$- \frac{Number\ of\ injured\ athletes\ in\ a\ season}{Number\ of\ athletes\ at\ risk\ of\ being\ injured\ in\ a\ season}_{unexposed}$$

If no difference exists, the resulting point estimate will be approximately 0, or a null association.[1,3] The point estimate from a difference measure is interpreted as, "the risk/rate of injury among the exposed is x percentage points greater/less than the risk/rate of injury among the unexposed." The advantage of the rate/risk difference over the rate/risk ratio is that it includes information about the scale of injury incidence, which is not represented in ratio measures. For example, a spine fracture may be 10 times as likely in one group than another; however, the incidence of spine fractures may be very low in both groups, which is important to know.[20] The risk difference provides this information, whereas the risk ratio does not.

When calculating these measures of injury occurrence and association from data, it is important to remember that these estimates are only as good as the sample from which they were calculated. In the case of rare events, it can be challenging to calculate stable estimates owing to small sample sizes and large standard errors. This factor should be considered in the study design phase and when interpreting results from analysis of small samples. Exact statistics are a class of statistics that are often more appropriate than regular (so-called "large sample") statistics when sample sizes are small. Exact statistics are particularly useful when the counts in some cells of analysis tables are very low (eg, ≤ 3).

MEASURES OF PHYSICAL PERFORMANCE AND TRAINING

Recent advances in technology have led to an increase in "wearable technologies" and the use of computer and video to measure functional movement. The goal of many of these technologies is to measure physical ability, workload, and fatigue in the hopes of predicting and implementing measures to mitigate injury. Given their relative recentness in the sports literature, especially in sports injury research, it is important to consider how to best use these measures in study designs and consider what these devices and metrics are actually measuring.

One of the most commonly used measures of training and workload are wearable global positioning software (GPS) devices, which track an athlete's heart rate, distance run, and intensity of work (time spent and distance run at different levels), among other things.[23] The goal is to use these measures to determine the amount of stress on the body, such that performance is maximized but risk of overtraining is minimized. These measures have been studied in research as both exposures (predictors of injury) and outcomes (as surrogates for fatigue and other performance measures).[24–27] This measure provides an objective counterpart to previously used subjective measures of training and effort, such as the rating of perceived exertion scale,[28] which has been associated with injury.[29] A particular area of emphasis has been acute workload (usually measured within the course of single conditioning session or competition or days) compared with chronic workload (usually measured over the course of weeks or an entire season) and the effect of the ratio of these measures on injury.[30,31] Evidence shows that moderate workloads, as well as a moderate acute:chronic workload ratio is protective of injury, and the ratio of acute:chronic workload may be more predictive of injury than workloads themselves, although much of this work has been done using subjective measures.[30,32–34]

In addition to measuring workload, these technologies can be used to measure exposure for risks and rates. If an athlete logs time on a GPS device, then the researcher knows that he or she participated in athletic activity for that day. This provides an athlete–exposure count, but it also allows for more detailed exposure measurement, such as player–minutes.

Subjective measures of functional movement, such as the Landing Error Scoring System and Balance Error Scoring System have long existed to predict injury or measure possible deficits in movement after injury.[35,36] Additionally, technology using force plates has been used to measure movement and balance. More recently, however, these measures have been integrated with video systems for motion capture. This includes formal systems designed for motion capture, as well as adaptations of existing video game systems for the purposes of measuring physical performance and functional movement.[37,38] These tools have been used to both predict injury and capture deficits in physical performance after injury.

STUDY DESIGN CONSIDERATIONS FOR MEASURES OF PHYSICAL PERFORMANCE

Although many of these measures of physical performance and training have been used in clinical situations and by coaches, especially strength and conditioning coaches, their use in research is still limited. Most studies have been done to validate the measures as predictors of injury or determine how the findings associate with other known measures of the same constructs. As use of these metrics become more widespread, researchers must consider study design implications. For example:

- Are these measures the exposure of interest or the outcome of interest? That is, is training load or functional movement leading to injury or game performance outcomes, or are other factors leading to training load or functional movement?
- Are the devices used measuring the construct of interest? And, more important, what is the construct of interest and why?
- How are these data aggregated across a game, season, or career? Are the average values most meaningful, or is the change in value over time more meaningful? How is a continuous stream of data analyzed and interpreted?
- What is the best way to measure "training load" or "fatigue"? As mentioned, recent research has examined whether acute, chronic or the ratio of acute:-chronic workload is most relevant. In addition to this, the definition of "acute" versus "chronic" varies across research studies. The GPS devices also provide a wide range of measures, including heart rate, distance run, to time in certain heart rate zones, number of sprints, and so on. Choosing the best measure is difficult and may depend on the research question. If all are used in separate analyses, researchers should consider the implications of performing so many comparisons surrounding the same research question.
- These data are often collected multiple times across the course of the season, often daily, on the same research subjects. As such, methods that account for multiple observations per subject, such as mixed models, should be used to ensure that assumptions of statistical independence associated with traditional statistical techniques are not violated.

SUMMARY

Although sports analytics have long been a part of sport, their use continues to grow, with emphasis on measuring sports injury and physical aptitude. Most existing epidemiologic and research study designs can be used in the sports setting, but there are special considerations that researchers must take and clinicians reading sports research studies should consider. In particular, researchers should carefully choose what measures of injury occurrence they plan to measure and how these data will be collected, what study design makes the most sense for the research question at hand, and how measures such as "recurrent injury" and "workload" will be defined. With these considerations in mind, a high-quality research study can provide valuable insights into injury prevention and management.

REFERENCES

1. Rothman KJ. Epidemiology: an introduction. 2nd edition. New York: Oxford University Press; 2012.
2. Bryant DM, Willits K, Hanson BP. Principles of designing a cohort study in orthopaedics. J Bone Joint Surg Am 2009;91(Suppl 3):10–4.
3. Rothman KJ, Greenland S, Lash TL. Modern epidemiology. 3rd edition. Philadelphia: Lippincott Williams & Wilkins; 2008.

4. Wacholder S. The case-control study as data missing by design: estimating risk differences. Epidemiology 1996;7(2):144–50.
5. Kooistra B, Dijkman B, Einhorn TA, et al. How to design a good case series. J Bone Joint Surg Am 2009;91(Suppl 3):21–6.
6. Ekegren CL, Gabbe BJ, Finch CF. Sports injury surveillance systems: a review of methods and data quality. Sports Med 2016;46(1):49–65.
7. Holder Y, Peden M, Krug E, et al. In: Holder Y, et al, editors. Injury surveillance guidelines. Geneva: World Health Organization; 2001. Available at: http://www.who.int/iris/handle/10665/42451.
8. Sports-related injuries among high school athletes–United States, 2005-06 school year. MMWR Morb Mortal Wkly Rep 2006;55(38):1037–40.
9. Valovich McLeod TC, Lam KC, Bay RC, et al. Practice-based research networks, part II: a descriptive analysis of the athletic training practice-based research network in the secondary school setting. J Athl Train 2012;47(5):557–66.
10. Dompier TP, Marshall SW, Kerr ZY, et al. The National Athletic Treatment, Injury and Outcomes Network (NATION): methods of the Surveillance Program, 2011-2012 Through 2013-2014. J Athl Train 2015;50(8):862–9.
11. Kerr ZY, Dompier TP, Snook EM, et al. National collegiate athletic association injury surveillance system: review of methods for 2004-2005 through 2013-2014 data collection. J Athl Train 2014;49(4):552–60.
12. Orchard JW, Seward H, Orchard JJ. Results of 2 decades of injury surveillance and public release of data in the Australian Football League. Am J Sports Med 2013;41(4):734–41.
13. Brooks JH, Fuller CW, Kemp SP, et al. Epidemiology of injuries in English professional rugby union: part 1 match injuries. Br J Sports Med 2005;39(10):757–66.
14. Pollack KM, D'Angelo J, Green G, et al. Developing and implementing major league baseball's health and injury tracking system. Am J Epidemiol 2016; 183(5):490–6.
15. National Athletic Trainers' Association. Recommendations and Guidelines for Appropriate Medical Coverage of Intercollegiate Athletics. Available at: https://www.nata.org/professional-interests/job-settings/college-university/resources/AMCIA. Accessed October 30, 2017.
16. van Mechelen W. Sports injury surveillance systems. 'One size fits all'? Sports Med 1997;24(3):164–8.
17. United States Consumer Product Safety Commission. National Electronic Injury Surveillance System (NEISS). Available at: https://www.cpsc.gov/Research–Statistics/NEISS-Injury-Data. Accessed March 6, 2018.
18. Brooks JH, Fuller CW, Kemp SP, et al. A prospective study of injuries and training amongst the England 2003 Rugby World Cup squad. Br J Sports Med 2005; 39(5):288–93.
19. Kerr ZY, Roos KG, Djoko A, et al. Epidemiologic measures for quantifying the incidence of concussion in national collegiate athletic association sports. J Athl Train 2017;52(3):167–74.
20. Knowles SB, Marshall SW, Guskiewicz KM. Issues in estimating risks and rates in sports injury research. J Athl Train 2006;41(2):207–15.
21. Finch CF, Cook J. Categorising sports injuries in epidemiological studies: the subsequent injury categorisation (SIC) model to address multiple, recurrent and exacerbation of injuries. Br J Sports Med 2014;48(17):1276–80.
22. Hamilton GM, Meeuwisse WH, Emery CA, et al. Subsequent injury definition, classification, and consequence. Clin J Sport Med 2011;21(6):508–14.

23. Coutts AJ, Duffield R. Validity and reliability of GPS devices for measuring movement demands of team sports. J Sci Med Sport 2010;13(1):133–5.
24. Ehrmann FE, Duncan CS, Sindhusake D, et al. GPS and injury prevention in professional Soccer. J Strength Cond Res 2016;30(2):360–7.
25. Mara JK, Thompson KG, Pumpa KL, et al. Periodization and physical performance in elite female soccer players. Int J Sports Physiol Perform 2015;10(5): 664–9.
26. Colby MJ, Dawson B, Heasman J, et al. Accelerometer and GPS-derived running loads and injury risk in elite Australian footballers. J Strength Cond Res 2014; 28(8):2244–52.
27. Bourdon PC, Cardinale M, Murray A, et al. Monitoring athlete training loads: consensus statement. Int J Sports Physiol Perform 2017;12(Suppl 2):S2161–70.
28. Foster C, Florhaug JA, Franklin J, et al. A new approach to monitoring exercise training. J Strength Cond Res 2001;15(1):109–15.
29. Gabbett TJ, Jenkins DG. Relationship between training load and injury in professional rugby league players. J Sci Med Sport 2011;14(3):204–9.
30. Malone S, Owen A, Newton M, et al. The acute:chronic workload ratio in relation to injury risk in professional soccer. J Sci Med Sport 2017;20(6):561–5.
31. Nassis GP, Gabbett TJ. Is workload associated with injuries and performance in elite football? A call for action. Br J Sports Med 2017;51(6):486–7.
32. Gabbett TJ. The training-injury prevention paradox: should athletes be training smarter and harder? Br J Sports Med 2016;50(5):273–80.
33. Malone S, Roe M, Doran D, et al. Protection against spikes in workload with aerobic fitness and playing experience: the role of the acute: chronic workload ratio on injury risk in elite Gaelic football. Int J Sports Physiol Perform 2017;12(3): 393–401.
34. Hulin BT, Gabbett TJ, Caputi P, et al. Low chronic workload and the acute:chronic workload ratio are more predictive of injury than between-match recovery time: a two-season prospective cohort study in elite rugby league players. Br J Sports Med 2016;50(16):1008–12.
35. Padua DA, Marshall SW, Boling MC, et al. The Landing Error Scoring System (LESS) is a valid and reliable clinical assessment tool of jump-landing biomechanics: the JUMP-ACL study. Am J Sports Med 2009;37(10):1996–2002.
36. Riemann BL, Guskiewicz KM. Effects of mild head injury on postural stability as measured through clinical balance testing. J Athl Train 2000;35(1):19–25.
37. Gray AD, Willis BW, Skubic M, et al. Development and validation of a portable and inexpensive tool to measure the drop vertical jump using the Microsoft Kinect V2. Sports Health 2017;9(6):537–44.
38. Merchant-Borna K, Jones CM, Janigro M, et al. Evaluation of Nintendo Wii balance board as a tool for measuring postural stability after sport-related concussion. J Athl Train 2017;52(3):245–55.

Mixed Methods Designs for Sports Medicine Research

Melissa C. Kay, MS, LAT, ATC*, Kristen L. Kucera, PhD, MSPH, LAT, ATC

KEYWORDS

- Mixed methodology • Qualitative • Quantitative • Sports medicine
- Research design

KEY POINTS

- Mixed methods research (MMR) encompasses the use of qualitative and quantitative methodological approaches to observe, evaluate, and understand particular phenomena of interest.
- MMR is adopted by researchers for a variety of reasons although the most important aspect is that using qualitative and quantitative techniques adds to topic understanding.
- The type of design selected for MMR should only be used if it is an appropriate approach driven by the research question.
- MMR does not simply encompass collecting 2 types of data but mixing the 2 procedures in an appropriate manner.
- MMR requires more time and resources than a single method in isolation, particularly if using a concurrent design where both methods are initiated simultaneously.

Mixed methods research (MMR) is a relatively new technique within sports medicine research where quantitative and qualitative research methods are combined. The purpose of this review is to detail 5 particular aspects of MMR, including (1) what MMR is, (2) when MMR should be used, (3) types of MMR designs, (4) how MMR has been used in sports medicine, and (5) considerations for future use of MMR within sports medicine. On conclusion of reading this review, readers should have a thorough understanding of the benefits MMR provides to the field of sports medicine moving forwards.

WHAT IS MIXED METHODS RESEARCH?

There are 2 primary types of research methods used within sports medicine currently: quantitative and qualitative. Quantitative research is primarily conducted via investigation of a particular research question and/or hypothesis, which generates numbers and uses statistical analyses to produce descriptive and inferential

Department of Exercise and Sport Science, Matthew Gfeller Sport-Related Traumatic Brain Injury Research Center, University of North Carolina at Chapel Hill, 209 Fetzer Hall, CB #8700, Chapel Hill, NC 27599, USA
* Corresponding author.
E-mail address: mkay@email.unc.edu

Clin Sports Med 37 (2018) 401–412
https://doi.org/10.1016/j.csm.2018.03.005
0278-5919/18/© 2018 Elsevier Inc. All rights reserved.

sportsmed.theclinics.com

statistics.[1] Most surveys and experimental studies use quantitative methods allowing for deductive reasoning. A hallmark of quantitative research is the consideration and emphasis on internal and external validity as well as reliability to ensure that results are repeatable and generalizable to the populations under investigation.[2] In turn, qualitative research is hypothesis generating meaning that nothing is predetermined and the focus is on gaining context or explanation of why or how a phenomenon exists.[3] Focus groups, key informant interviews, and open-ended surveys are examples of qualitative research that allow for inductive reasoning. As quantitative focuses on validity and reliability for rigor, qualitative research has its own methods of establishing strength. Instead of reliability, qualitative data use the concepts of consistency and trustworthiness whereas validity incorporates correctness, strength, and credibility of statements being given.[4–6] Sport medicine researchers tend to use these methods in isolation, which may be appropriate given the research questions under study. By using these methods individually, however, researchers may not be getting a full picture of phenomena that exist.

MMR is defined as "the type of research in which a researcher or team of researchers combines elements of qualitative and quantitative research approaches for the broad purposes of breadth and depth of understanding and corroboration."[4] Specifically, quantitative and qualitative approaches are combined in at least one way during a single study via techniques, methods, or concepts.[4–7] MMR is particularly useful for phenomena in which there are multiple stakeholders or influencing factors. This design allows for further context and meaning to be provided to statistical information, which often carries a great deal of weight with readers. In the field of sports medicine, an example of this multidisciplinary care is related to concussive injuries, such as barriers to incorporating academic accommodations after injury, under-reporting of injuries, and removing an individual from participation, which all require the collaboration of multiple stakeholders.

WHEN TO USE MIXED METHODS RESEARCH DESIGNS

When identifying which research method is most appropriate for use, researchers consider the specific research question and the population under study. Although this is necessary for any design being selected, it is imperative for use in MMR due to the variety of design sequences that exist.[8–11] The decision to use an MMR design lies solely in the additional value given to findings by using both qualitative and quantitative methods together as opposed to in isolation[5,12] (**Box 1**). This lends itself to research problems and questions that are multifaceted in nature with multiple viewpoints or perspectives on a problem that need to be considered as parts of a whole.[9,13–15] Despite the large benefit this provides to researchers, it also is a source

---

Box 1
Key characteristics of mixed methods research

- Incorporates the use of qualitative and quantitative research methods[4–7,14]
  - Requires mixing of the 2 procedures, not simply collecting both types of information

- Adopted for 5 primary reasons[6,17,18]:
  - Triangulation/corroboration of different findings within one phenomenon
  - Complementary to enhance or clarify results from one method to another
  - Initiation to discover a new process or perspective
  - Development of one method from another method's results
  - Expansion of findings from one method to provide context to another

of burden. There are many benefits to answering the research question; however, MMR requires additional skills and collaboration of the research team as well as time and resources because 2 studies are essentially performed simultaneously (**Table 1**).[16]

There are 5 primary reasons why a researcher would want to adopt MMR for a research study, including (1) triangulation/corroboration, (2) complementarity, (3) initiation, (4) development, and (5) expansion.[6,17,18] These reasons are specific to MMR compared with qualitative or quantitative research in isolation. Triangulation (or corroboration) is characterized by converging results from both methods to study the same research question or phenomenon. Triangulation proposes to increase the validity of the findings because one method is used to reinsure the other. Complementarity refers to the enhancement or elaboration of results from one method with the results from another to answer complementary research questions or multiple pieces of the same phenomenon. Complementarity is proposed to increase the validity of results by providing contextual interpretation or meaning. Initiation is used to discover or explore new perspectives or ideas about a previously studied phenomenon. Initiation increases breadth and depth of the results being studied. Development occurs when one method is needed to develop the other method. This is a sequential method by nature because the first method is necessary to shape not only data collection but also sampling and analysis of the next phase. Development is used to increase the validity of results, particularly when a phenomenon is not as well understood. Lastly, expansion uses multiple methods to study multiple phenomenon that may be interrelated increasing the breadth and scope of analysis.

A researcher may have one reason or multiple for adopting MMR; regardless, it is important to consider the strengths of qualitative and quantitative methods individually to ensure they complement each other within MMR and reduce the weaknesses associated with each.[1] Quantitative phases can provide statistical power and broad generalizability while qualitative phases ensure meaning, context, and depth imperative to translation and implementation of research findings. When both methods are used and offset the flaws of one another, validity is enhanced.[17] For example, Smith and colleagues[19] designed a randomized controlled trial for patellofemoral pain that was created based on qualitative research to understand an injury's effect on participants daily life. Participants were enrolled in a quantitative randomized controlled trial and completed the intervention. A subset of participants completed a postintervention qualitative interview to discuss the acceptability and feasibility of the intervention. The benefit MMR provided to this study included highlighting the strengths of patient care via a randomized controlled trial while also allowing for context and meaning that may influence the implementation of this method within clinical practice. Even though

Table 1
Benefits and challenges of mixed methods research

Benefits	Challenges
• Allows for deeper understanding of a problem[14,25]	• Requires significant time, planning, resources,[16,20] and personnel[5,16,26,27]
• Compatible methods for the purpose of answering specific research questions[17,28,29]	• Some individuals do not see benefit,[4] making it difficult to publish results together.
• Flexibility to assess and understand a phenomenon not easily addressed by one method in isolation[9,13]	• Potential for contradictory findings[21,22]

the strengths of MMR are vast, there are opponents and challengers who express the differences in paradigms, thereby nullifying the combination of methods.[4–7] These opponents make the claim that the 2 approaches cannot be combined due to the differences in thought processes making the dissemination of results difficult. Therefore, it is imperative to provide readers with a thorough explanation of why the researchers chose to use MMR within articles.

There are several challenges that exist regarding the implementation of MMR applications (see **Table 1**). First, MMR incorporates 2 phases, which may occur simultaneously or in succession. Regardless, having 2 phases of the research process that require extra planning, time, and funding prevent many researchers from using MMR.[16,20] Second, because data collection is from 2 separate methods, it is possible to receive contradictory findings or findings that are unexpected. Often, this does not come to light until the study has already been initiated, making it difficult for researchers to interpret or move forward.[21,22] Lastly, MMR has a stigma with other researchers who believe only quantitative or only qualitative research methods produce legitimate claims.[4] This challenge puts mixed methods researchers in a difficult position where they often must discuss qualitative and quantitative findings separately.[23,24] Ironically, this challenge provides a strong platform for mixed methods researchers to introduce single-method researchers to the unique benefit MMR provides.[20]

MIXED METHODS STUDY DESIGNS

As with any research study, the predetermined questions drive all pieces from conception to design to data collection and analysis in MMR; however, because there are multiple phases and multiple methods, it is important to have separate questions or aims related to the qualitative and quantitative portions.[1,18,30–32] Once the research questions have been formulated, a researcher has 3 important decisions to make. The first decision is in regard to separation of the qualitative and quantitative phases. These phases can run either sequentially or concurrently and the way in which they are completed is determined by the research questions.[20] For sequential phases, it is nearly impossible to keep the 2 phases separate because one builds on the other, whereas in concurrent phases, they can be kept separate until the end because the 2 phases do not influence each other during the process. For example, Barton and colleagues[33] used an explanatory sequential study where quantitative data was gathered via a literature review followed by clinician interviews to explain why these techniques are chosen to treat lower extremity injuries in runners. An example of the concurrent option is shown via a different study by Barton and colleagues[34] on patellofemoral pain management. In this study, data were collected concurrently meaning that one type did not influence the other. The second decision is about whether or not a researcher is going to place emphasis on the qualitative or quantitative portion or treat them as equals. Sequential studies typically place weight whereas concurrent studies do not. For example, in explanatory sequential designs, like the one discussed previously, weight is placed on the quantitative portion because that is the first part conducted to gather data on a well-known phenomenon. In exploratory sequential designs, the weight is on the qualitative information to truly understand and explore a lesser known phenomenon to design and gather quantitative data. The final decision determines when mixing of the 2 methods will occur. Mixed methods does not simply use the collection of data from 2 different methods but also connects them in some way, shape, or form, to draw conclusions about a research problem. The mixing between the 2 methods can occur at any stage in the research process; however, it is critical to performing true MMR.[10,35] There are 3 primary ways mixing occurs (integration, connection, and embedding), although they do not have to be used in isolation.[5,35] Integration is used when qualitative and quantitative data are collected concurrently, analyzed separately, and then integrated during interpretation. In a study conducted by Crowther and colleagues,[36] they used a concurrent design to collect qualitative and quantitative data on recovery strategies used for athletes. This required them to keep data separate until the end where findings were integrated. Connection occurs when one approach is based on findings from another, meaning collection occurs sequentially to build on one another. Chinn and Porter[37] used connection for their mixing method when completing an explanatory sequential study on concussion knowledge and reporting behaviors to connect qualitative to initial quantitative findings. This type of design allowed the researchers to take initial analyses a step further and actually explain why their participants had particular knowledge and reporting behaviors. The connection between the 2 types of data meant researchers could draw conclusions using both aspects. Embedding is when the mixing is throughout the entire process by implanting one type (typically qualitative) into a study of another type (typically quantitative). For example, in a study completed by Sandal and colleagues,[38] an embedded design was used by conducting focus groups with each type of participant (control vs experimental) during a randomized controlled trial to optimize treatment delivery for those who had been waitlisted to the intervention. By conducting focus groups with the first experimental group, the research team was able to refine the intervention and optimize delivery to the waitlisted group. This ability would be lost within just a quantitative study.

These features are all pieces of 4 specific types of study designs, which are conducted for different reasons, including concurrent (also known as convergent or parallel),[34,36,39–41] exploratory sequential, explanatory sequential,[37,42] or embedded (also known as nested) (**Table 2**).[38] The concurrent MMR design is used to gain different, albeit complementary, data to answer a single research question. The qualitative and quantitative phases are conducted simultaneously and are weighted equally.[7,20] In the exploratory sequential design, the qualitative phase is conducted first, followed by the quantitative. It is typically used for research problems which are not yet well understood and allow for the quantitative study to be built on the qualitative findings. Exploratory sequential is qualitative dominant because it is central to understanding a population or a problem prior to initiating the quantitative portion.[5] Explanatory sequential is just the opposite. Quantitative data are conducted first followed by the qualitative phase to allow for elaboration or context of the findings and the quantitative phase becomes dominant.[5] Lastly, an embedded design can place weight on either the qualitative or quantitative portion and is typically dictated by a researcher's specialty. This type is used to collect different data for different, yet complementary, research questions where one method is nested within the other.[42]

MIXED METHODS IN SPORTS MEDICINE

Sports medicine research frequently faces problems needing to be addressed by encompassing both the science behind a construct as well as the implementation of said science. Often, accomplishing both of these tasks is not possible with a single approach.[21] As such, it is important that sports medicine researchers adopt a more holistic approach, including quantitative and qualitative methodology, to answering the problems faced by clinicians in the field. Just because mixed methods designs may be appropriate for inclusion in sports medicine research as a whole, however, it may not be applicable to every single research study undertaken by an individual.

Table 2
Types of mixed methods research designs with corresponding prioritization and benefits

Design Type	Definition/Sequence	Dominance	Benefit of Use

Concurrent
• Also known as
  ○ Convergent
  ○ Parallel
	Qualitative and quantitative processes occur simultaneously	Equal weight between qualitative and quantitative	Can obtain data that are different, yet complementary, to address a single research question[7,20]
			Add credibility to findings[21]

Exploratory sequential	Qualitative then quantitative	Qualitative dominant	Useful for studying issues that are not yet well understood[5] Increases generalizability by quantitative building on qualitative findings[5]
Explanatory sequential	Quantitative then qualitative	Quantitative dominant	Qualitative data add context and meaning to initial findings that are more rigid.[5]
Embedded • Also known as nested	Quantitative within qualitative study OR Qualitative within quantitative study	Qualitative or quantitative Whichever process is being embedded is the less dominant method	Used to answer complementary research questions that would benefit from both types of research design, although may not require an entirely separate methodological focus[42]

Of the 4 primary types of MMR designs listed previously, it is imperative to look at the particular characteristics of these designs in combination with the proposed research questions of any project. MMR should only be used if it adds value to the project as a whole.[5,12] Even more so, it is necessary to preemptively decide how the MMR will be conducted from start to finish, including design type, data collection, data analyses, and the mixing of qualitative and quantitative information.[5,35] Albeit new, mixed methods have been used by sports medicine researchers successfully. Researchers must not simply collect 2 types of data but also allow for the incorporation of data to enhance findings and conclusions. Without this crucial step, sports medicine researchers are not actually conducting true MMR; therefore. the benefit of MMR is lost, including connecting the dots between findings. One example of this is the ability of Sandal and colleagues[38] to optimize treatment delivery for a waitlisted group by learning the perceptions of initial participants. Without the focus group, the waitlisted group would have received the exact same intervention with no refinement. **Table 3** outlines how MMR has been used by sports medicine researchers until this point, including the topic it was used to address, the specific design type used, the reason they adopted MMR, and how they chose to mix the 2 types of data.

Table 3
Mixed methods research in sports medicine research: examples from the literature

Author	Topic	Design	Reason for Adoption	Mixing Method
Barton et al,[34] 2015	Patellofemoral pain conservative management techniques	Concurrent: literature review (quantitative) was conducted with concurrent patient and expert interviews (qualitative), analyzed separately, then combined	Triangulation of expert and patient perspectives with recent literature to determine best management approaches for patellofemoral pain	Integration: kept separate until data analysis and then merged to aid in interpretation of findings
Chinn & Porter,[37] 2016	Concussion knowledge and reporting behaviors	Explanatory sequential: quantitative survey data were collected prior to qualitative interviews to understand concussion education and how it has an impact on the reporting of concussions.	Complementarity of concussion knowledge with the lack of reporting behavior despite being educated	Connection: the quantitative data are used as a foundation of concussion knowledge and behavior whereas qualitative data help explain or understand said behaviour.
Crowther et al,[36] 2017	Postexercise recovery techniques used by athletes	Concurrent: qualitative and quantitative data were collected in parallel via a single survey featuring close-ended and open-ended questions, analyzed separately, then combined.	Triangulation of the patient perspective on recovery methods used by team sport athletes	Integration: kept separate until data analysis and then merged to aid in interpretation of findings
Granquist et al,[39] 2014	Rehabilitation adherence in athletic training	Concurrent: qualitative and quantitative data were collected in parallel via a single survey featuring close-ended and open-ended questions, analyzed separately, then combined.	Complementarity of athletic trainer perspective with rehabilitation adherence and the factors contributing to nonadherence in collegiate student-athletes	Integration: kept separate until data analysis and then merged to aid in interpretation of findings

(continued on next page)

Table 3
(continued)

Author	Topic	Design	Reason for Adoption	Mixing Method
Joseph et al,[40] 2014	Use of a triage system for musculoskeletal conditions	Concurrent: qualitative focus groups and a quantitative literature review were collected in parallel, analyzed separately, then combined.	Triangulation of expert and patient perspectives with recent literature to determine best approaches for triage system use for musculoskeletal conditions	Integration: kept separate until data analysis and then merged to aid in interpretation of findings
Rowe et al,[43] 2012	Clinical reasoning of Achilles tendinopathy management	Explanatory sequential: literature review (quantitative) was conducted to review evidence related to the management of Achilles tendinopathy followed by qualitative interviews related to how and why they choose which management route to take.	Complementarity of recent literature with the provider perspective to determine how and why particular management strategies are useful for Achilles tendinopathy	Connection: the evidence is used as a foundation to expert opinion of clinical reasoning for Achilles tendinopathy management.
Sandal et al,[38] 2017	Effect of physical environment on treatment and patient outcomes	Embedded: qualitative focus group interviews within a quantitative randomized controlled trial	Expansion of patient perspective on treatment delivery	Embedding: throughout entire project due to qualitative being within the quantitative
Turner et al,[41] 2017	Health literacy and knowledge of parents in youth sport leagues regarding concussion	Concurrent: qualitative interviews and quantitative survey data were collected in parallel, analyzed separately, then combined.	Triangulation of parent knowledge and literacy to reinsure findings of each method independently	Integration: kept separate until data analysis and then merged to aid in interpretation of findings

Overall, mixed methods have been used sparingly thus far within the field of sports medicine and athlete care. As shown in **Table 3**, there are only a few topics that have taken advantage of what MMR has to offer, including clinical reasoning and management techniques from a clinician perspective,[34,39,40,42] concussion knowledge and reporting,[37,41] and patient outcomes.[36,38] Few studies have explored injury in this manner apart from concussion or the clinician perspective, although this is a strong approach for injury experience and returning to participation from the patient perspective.

MMR has been used in limited topics of sports medicine research as well as the limited use of design and reasoning types. No published studies to date have used an exploratory sequential approach and there has only been limited use of the embedded design.[38] The exploratory sequential approach is a great step for many sports medicine researchers of topics that are less well known or still novel in concept, such as long-term effects of head impact exposure or emergency response and medical care surrounding catastrophic sport-related injury. The combination of patient experience, fear, and other factors along with the objective risk factor and outcome variables that exist allow for the development of novel conclusions connecting the clinician/patient with the researcher perspective.

Of the 5 main reasons for conducting qualitative research, only 3 were found in sports medicine for this review: triangulation,[34,36,40,41] complementarity,[37,39,43] and expansion.[38] This leaves initiation and development as potentially novel techniques and reasoning behind using MMR in sports medicine. These can be used to establish new links between phenomena and develop appropriate interventions to address a particular issue. For example, in the realm of athlete retirement, until research understands and shows how retirement affects athletes' daily life, social support, and other factors, an appropriate and effective preemptive intervention to prevent these issues on retirement cannot be designed.

CONSIDERATIONS FOR USING MIXED METHODS RESEARCH

It is important for researchers interested in conducting MMR in the field of sports medicine to consider applying these designs and approaches to novel areas of study that would benefit from a more holistic approach. For example, in a study of catastrophic sport injury recovery, researchers must consider not only the school or sport organization perspective but also the clinician, athlete, and parent perspective as well as true objective deficits after the injury. MMR could be used to better understand and approach all aspects of injury prevention, recognition, management, and return to the playing field. It is also important for interested researchers to consider the amount of resources required for conducting MMR properly. This is seldom a solo endeavor and requires the establishment of a qualified team with a broad range of skills, including qualitative, quantitative, and/or mixed methodological experiences.[5,16,26,27] Sports medicine research has primarily been driven by quantitative methodologies, which may produce hesitation by some for using MMR. Recent emphasis on interdisciplinary research and collaboration may improve knowledge surrounding qualitative as well as MMR methodologies. Even though MMR provides a wide range of benefits previously discussed, it is not an easy method to use and must be conducted with careful consideration of the feasibility and appropriateness to the research question. The field of sports medicine can greatly benefit from researchers using MMR to explore and explain sport injury and recovery because it is a field based in interdisciplinary and multiperspective care.

MMR requires more time and resources than a standard study, because essentially 2 studies are conducted at once. Because of this, interested researchers must prepare

---

Box 2
Key considerations for applying mixed methods research

- MMR requires more time and resources than conducting a qualitative or quantitative study in isolation.[5,16,20,26,27]

- MMR must be used only if it is a logical approach to the research question(s).[5]
  - The type of design must also mimic questions.

- MMR has received skepticism from individuals who think only qualitative or only quantitative research has value.[4]
  - It is important to keep the audience in mind as MMR is designed and implemented.

---

themselves in advance by assembling a strong research team as a critical first step. The next step requires thinking about the order of qualitative and quantitative data collection and what specific benefit each type of research is providing to the overall question. Although MMR is a relatively new technique within sports medicine research, it has a unique ability to provide perspective to aid in implementation of future findings.

The purpose of this review is to detail 5 particular aspects of MMR, including (1) what MMR is, (2) when MMR should be used, (3) types of MMR designs, (4) how MMR has been used in sports medicine, and (5) considerations for future use of MMR (**Box 2**). Readers should now have a thorough understanding of the benefits MMR provides to the field of sports medicine moving forward.

REFERENCES

1. Teddlie C, Tashakkori A. Foundations of mixed methods research. Integrating quantitative and qualitative approaches in the social and behavioral sciences. Thousand Oaks (CA): SAGE Publications; 2009.
2. Bowling A. Research methods in health. investigating health and health services. 3rd edition. Maidenhead (United Kingdom): Open University Press; 2009.
3. Pyett P. Validation of qualitative research in the "real world". Qual Health Res 2003;13(8):1170–9.
4. Johnson R, Onwuegbuzie A. Mixed methods research: a research paradigm whose time has come. Educational Researcher 2004;33(7):14–26.
5. Creswell JW, Plano-Clark V. Designing and conducting mixed methods research. 2nd edition. Thousand Oaks (CA): SAGE Publications; 2011.
6. Wisdom JP, Cavaleri MA, Onwuegbuzie A, et al. Methodological reporting in qualitative, quantitative, and mixed methods health services research articles. Health Serv Res 2012;47(2):721–45.
7. Halcomb E, Hickman L. Mixed methods research. Nurs Stand 2015;29(32):41–7.
8. McEvoy P, Richards D. A critical realist rationale for using a combination of quantitative and qualitative methods. J Res Nurs 2006;11(1):66–78.
9. Simons L, Lathlean J. Mixed methods. In: Gerrish K, Lacey A, editors. The research process in nursing. 6th edition. Oxford (United Kingdom): Wiley Blackwell; 2010. p. 331–44.
10. Glogowska M. Paradigms, pragmatism and possibilities: mixed-methods research in speech and language therapy. Int J Lang Commun Disord 2011; 46(3):251–60.
11. Maudsley G. Mixing it but not mixed-up: mixed methods research in medical education (a critical narrative review). Med Teach 2011;33(2):e92–104.

12. Scammon DL, Tomoaia-Cotisel A. Connecting the dots and merging meaning using mixed methods to study primary care delivery transformation. Health Serv Res 2013;48(6):2181–207.
13. Andrew S, Halcomb EJ. Mixed methods research. In: Borbasi S, Jackson D, editors. Navigating the maze of research: enhancing nursing and midwifery practice. 3rd edition. Marrickville (Australia): Elsevier; 2012. p. 147–66.
14. Burke Johnson R, Onwuegbuzie A, Turner L. Towards a definition of mixed methods research. J Mix Methods Res 2007;1:112–33.
15. Mason J. Real life methods: six strategies for mixing methods and linking data in social science research. Manchester (United Kingdom): University of Manchester; 2006.
16. Halcomb EJ, Andrew S. Practical considerations for higher degree research students undertaking mixed methods projects. International Journal of Multiple Research Approaches 2009;3(2):153–62.
17. Greene JC, Caracelli VJ, Graham WF. Toward a conceptual framework for mixed-methods evaluation. Educ Eval Policy Anal 1989;11(3):255–74.
18. Bryman A. Integrating quantitative and qualitative research: how is it done? Qualitative Research 2006;6(1):97–113.
19. Smith BE, Hendrick P, Bateman M, et al. Study protocol: a mixed methods feasibility study for a loaded self-managed exercise programme for patellofemoral pain. Pilot Feasibility Stud 2018;4:24.
20. van Griensven H, Moore AP, Hall V. Mixed methods research - the best of both worlds? Man Ther 2014;19:367–71.
21. Morgan D. Practical strategies for combining qualitative and quantitative methods: applications to health research. Qual Health Res 1998;8(3):362–76.
22. Brannen J. Mixing methods: the entry of qualitative and quantitative approaches into the research process. Int J Soc Res Methodol 2005;8(3):173–84.
23. Bryman A. Barriers to integrating quantitative and qualitative. J Mix Methods Res 2007;1(1):8–22.
24. Feilzer M. Doing mixed methods research pragmatically: implications for the rediscovery of pragmatism as a research paradigm. J Mix Methods Res 2010;4(1): 6–16.
25. Greene J. Mixing methods in social enquiry. San Francisco (CA): Wiley; 2007.
26. Bowers B, Cohen LW, Elliot AE, et al. Creating and supporting a mixed methods health services research team. Health Serv Res 2013;48(6):2157–80.
27. Lavelle E, Vuk J, Barber C. Twelve tips for getting started using mixed methods in medical education research. Med Teach 2013;35(4):272–6.
28. Rocco TS, Bliss LA, Gallagher S, et al. Taking the next step: mixed methods research in organizational systems. Information Technology, Learning, and Performance Journal 2003;21(1):19–29.
29. Petter SC, Gallivan MJ. Toward a framework for classifying and guiding mixed methods research in information system. In: Proceedings of the 37th Hawaii International Conference on System Science. Big Island, HI, January 5-8, 2004. p. 1–10.
30. Onwuegbuzie A, Johnson R. The validity issue in mixed research. Res Sch 2006; 13(1):48–63.
31. Greene J. Is mixed methods social inquiry a distinctive methodology? J Mix Methods Res 2008;2(1):7–22.
32. Creswell JW. Qualitative inquiry and research design. 2nd edition. Thousand Oaks (CA): SAGE Publications; 2007.

33. Barton CJ, Bonanno DR, Carr J, et al. Running retraining to treat lower limb injuries: a mixed-methods study of current evidence synthesised with expert opinion. Br J Sports Med 2016;50:513–26.

34. Barton CJ, Lack S, Hemmings S, et al. The "best practice guide to conservative management of patellofemoral pain": incorporating level 1 evidence with expert clinical reasoning. Br J Sports Med 2015;49:923–34.

35. Zhang W, Creswell JW. The use of "mixing" procedure of mixed methods in health services research. Med Care 2013;51(8):e51–7.

36. Crowther F, Sealey R, Crowe M, et al. Team sport athletes' perceptions and use of recovery strategies: a mixed-methods survey study. BMC Sports Sci Med Rehabil 2017;9(6):1–16.

37. Chinn NR, Porter P. Concussion reporting behaviours of community college student-athletes and limits of transferring concussion knowledge during the stress of competition. BMJ Open Sport Exerc Med 2016;2(1):e000118.

38. Sandal LF, Thorlund JB, Moore AJ, et al. Room for improvement: a randomised controlled trial with nested qualitative interviews on space, place and treatment delivery. Br J Sports Med 2017;1–9.

39. Granquist MD, Podlog L, Engel JR, et al. Certified athletic trainers' perspectives on rehabilitation adherence in collegiate athletic training settings. J Sport Rehabil 2014;23:123–33.

40. Joseph C, Morrissey D, Abdur-Rahman M, et al. Musculoskeletal triage: a mixed methods study, integrating systematic review with expert and patient perspectives. Physiotherapy 2014;100:277–89.

41. Turner RW, Lucas JW, Margolis LH, et al. A preliminary study of youth sport concussions: parents' health literacy and knowledge of return-to-play protocol criteria. Brain Inj 2017;31(8):1124–30.

42. Plano-Clark V, Schumacher K, West C, et al. Practices for embedding an interpretative qualitative approach within a randomized clinical trial. J Mix Methods Res 2013;7(3):219–42.

43. Rowe V, Hemmings S, Barton C, et al. Conservative management of midportion achilles tendinopathy. Sports Med 2012;42(11):941–67.

Considerations and Interpretation of Sports Injury Prevention Studies

Saulo Delfino Barboza, MSc[a], Roland Rössler, PhD[a,b],
Evert Verhagen, PhD[a,c],*

KEYWORDS

- Athletic injuries • Sports medicine • Epidemiologic methods • Injury prevention

KEY POINTS

- Study designs on sports injury prevention are prospective by default, and clinicians should consider the external validity of findings before applying preventative measures in their context.
- Injuries and injury rates should not be the sole outcome of injury prevention studies while outcomes of injury prevention efforts are also measurable in terms of severity, burden, and compliance/adherence to preventative strategies.
- Sports injury prevention studies should provide a clear definition of what was considered an injury in the study, data on sport exposure, severity of injury, and compliance/adherence to preventative measures.

INTRODUCTION

Maintaining a physically active lifestyle is a major contemporary public health issue.[1] Therefore, promoting sport participation is crucial for contemporary society.[2] The paradox is that, on the one hand, sport participation improves health through the well-documented benefits of regular physical exercise.[3] On the other hand, sport participation also increases the risk of unfavorable consequences, such as sports injuries.[4] The negative experience associated with injuries can discourage maintaining sport participation, which conflicts public health efforts.[2] Moreover, sports injuries negatively

The authors have no conflicts of interest to disclose.
[a] Amsterdam Collaboration on Health and Safety in Sports, Department of Public and Occupational Health, Amsterdam Public Health Research Institute, VU University Medical Center, Van der Boechorststraat 7, Amsterdam 1081 BT, The Netherlands; [b] Department of Sport, Exercise and Health, University of Basel, Birsstrasse 320 B, Basel 4052, Switzerland; [c] Division of Exercise Science and Sports Medicine, University of Cape Town, Anzio Road, Observatory, Cape Town 7925, South Africa
* Corresponding author. Amsterdam Collaboration on Health and Safety in Sports, Department of Public and Occupational Health, Amsterdam Public Health research institute, VU University Medical Center, Van der Boechorststraat 7, Amsterdam 1081 BT, The Netherlands.
E-mail address: e.verhagen@vumc.nl

Clin Sports Med 37 (2018) 413–425
https://doi.org/10.1016/j.csm.2018.03.006
0278-5919/18/© 2018 Elsevier Inc. All rights reserved.

influence team and individual athletic success.[5] Given the detrimental impact of sports injuries for the individual and society, preventative efforts are of great importance.[6]

Through understanding of research methodology, clinicians are better able to assess whether a research finding is valid and applicable for their context. Accordingly, this article is meant to be a resource for sport clinicians to understand and interpret (1) study design, (2) outcome measures, and (3) statistics in sports injuries prevention research. This should provide a foundation of knowledge for clinicians on the decision-making process to apply research findings in the area of injury prevention in practice.

STUDY DESIGNS IN INJURY PREVENTION STUDIES

Sports injuries prevention efforts follow, in general, the sequence of prevention (**Fig. 1**).[7] The extent of the injury problem should first be established (step 1) and subsequently the problem's underlying etiology and mechanisms investigated (step 2). After following these first 2 steps, there should be enough information to develop and introduce a preventative strategy (step 3) and, finally, assess its (cost-) effectiveness (step 4). This article focuses on the methodology of step 4 of the sequence of prevention, that is, assessing the (cost-) effectiveness of an injury prevention strategy.

There needs to be a clear distinction between efficacy and effectiveness of preventative measures. Efficacy describes the effect of any intervention under fully controlled and ideal conditions, taking any potential disturbing factors into account and giving the intervention the best conditions to demonstrate a beneficial effect. This is usually done in explanatory randomized controlled trials (RCTs)[8] and gives an answer to the

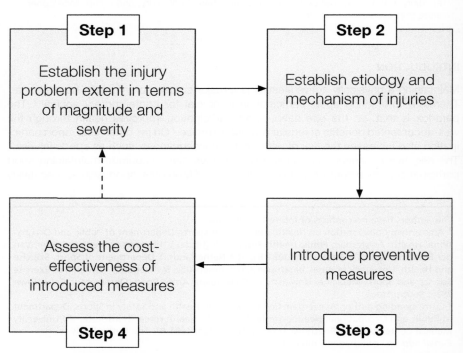

Fig. 1. The sequence of prevention of sports injury. (*Adapted from* van Mechelen W, Hlobil H, Kemper HCG. Incidence, severity, aetiology and prevention of sports injuries. Sports Med 1992;14(2):84; with permission.)

question, "Does the intervention work under ideal circumstances?"[9] Effectiveness is established under less controlled, more pragmatic conditions.[10] As such, the outcomes are more influenced by external factors that act in a true sports context. This type of outcome stems usually from less controlled study designs and answers the question, "Does the intervention work in a real-world context?"[9] Naturally, efficacy of a developed intervention should first be established before moving to effectiveness trials followed by implementation.

Randomized Controlled Trials

The efficacy of an injury prevention strategy is investigated through an RCT; this is the most rigorous design to infer a cause-effect relationship between a preventative strategy (ie, the intervention) and injury occurrence (ie, the outcome).[11] In an RCT, a randomization process allocates study participants to at least 2 groups: an intervention (eg, the group exposed to the preventative strategy) and a control group (eg, the group not exposed to the preventative strategy). Both groups are then followed over a preset period of time (eg, 1 season). The randomization process accounts for potential differences between participants' characteristics that might influence their response to the intervention and their baseline risk of injury. Therefore, in a well-conducted RCT, researchers can assume that known and unknown participants' characteristics are similar in both the intervention and control groups, and the intervention is virtually the only difference between both groups.[11]

An RCT, as discussed previously, usually assumes that each individual is an independent unit. In sports this is not always the case. Many sports are practiced in teams, and the issue is confronted that entire teams need to be randomized to an intervention or control group (ie, a cluster RCT). As an example, a cluster RCT investigated the effect of a structured warm-up program on the rate of injuries in young soccer players from different countries, clubs, and teams.[12] Clubs were randomized to intervention and a control groups, that is, structured warm-up and usual session, respectively. Clubs were randomized into the same group to minimize the risk of contamination (ie, participants of the control group knowing about and adopting the intervention). Country, age group, and number of participating teams per club served as strata for the randomization.

Beyond Randomized Controlled Trials

There are also several limitations to RCTs.[11] In sports injuries prevention research, it is argued that the main issue is its validity. Given the well-controlled study design, RCTs have high internal validity—results can be very trustable inside the specific controlled setting in which the study was conducted. RCTs often lack external validity also due to the well-controlled study design[13]—an efficacious preventative measure may not work as expected when applied in a setting that differs from the one originally studied. Therefore, nonrandomized study designs are also valid to evaluate the effectiveness of an efficacious preventative strategy in less controlled, real-life situations.[14]

Nonrandomized studies are considered a group of study designs that lack random allocation of participants to intervention and control group.[15] In sports injuries prevention, those include non-RCTs (ie, quasi-experiments) and prospective cohort studies, which can be experimental (ie, with an intervention) or not (ie, observational).[14] Prospective experimental cohorts, or pretest–post-test designs, enable time-trend analysis to evaluate injury rates before and after the implementation of preventative measures. This approach is useful for evaluating the effect of, for example, sporting rule changes aimed at reducing injuries[16] and nationwide injury prevention campaigns.[17] Prospective observational cohort studies may be used to monitor injury occurence and investigate the effect of preventative strategies already in use. For example, a study monitored ice hockey players who had been wearing full-face shields and players wearing half-face shields over a season.[18] This study found that ice hockey players wearing full-face shields had a lower injury risk of facial and dental injuries and recommended that the sport governing body should consider mandating full-facial protective gear.

The lack of random allocation in nonrandomized studies potentially leads to systematic differences between the groups studied[11]; therefore, the nonrandom allocation bias should be considered when inferring a cause-effect relationship between a preventative strategy and injury occurence in nonrandomized studies. For this reason, nonrandomized studies have lower internal validity than RCTs.[15] On the other hand, nonrandomized studies have more potential to emulate real-world experiences when applying research findings and, therefore, have increased external validity.[19]

OUTCOME MEASURES IN INJURY PREVENTION STUDIES

When studying the effect of injury preventative efforts, multiple outcomes need to be assessed to provide reliable results and meaningful conclusions. Naturally, injury is the main outcome of interest. The constructs exposure, severity, and compliance or adherence are also key elements to establish the outcome of injury preventative efforts.

Injury

The issue of defining what is a recordable sports injury in epidemiologic studies has been investigated comprehensively.[20] There are strict as well as broad injury definitions available. Definitions of injury can be summarized as injuries that lead to sport time loss, injuries that require medical attention, or all complaints that are reported by athletes.[20] The sport time loss definition, by default, concentrates on more severe injuries because athletes may continue participation in training and competition despite having a minor injury.[21] A time-loss injury does not necessarily receive medical attention because this is highly dependent on medical staff availability. In some cases, injured athletes may not consult health professionals. For example, a field hockey player could sustain a contusion in the thigh during a collision with another player. This contusion could lead to 1 or more days of time loss, without the player considering medical care. The medical attention definition, however, enables capturing injuries regardless of sport time loss. The all complaints definition enables capturing injuries beyond medical attention and time loss and also allows for more frequent monitoring of health complaints (**Fig. 2**). There are also studies focusing on the prevention of specific injuries (eg, anterior cruciate ligament or hamstring injuries), which, by default, have a specific definition of a recordable injury and its appropriate diagnosis.

Although standardized definitions in sports injuries research facilitate comparability between different studies and data pooling for meta-analyses, the chosen definition should reflect the goals of the study and the context of the surveillance. Clinicians should consider the strengths and limitations of each approach while interpreting findings on sports injuries prevention research.[20]

Sport Exposure

Measuring the number of injuries is fundamental in sports injuries prevention studies. Data on the exposure to sport are also essential, however, to provide some context to the actual risk of sustaining an injury while participating in sports.[22] If investigating the effectiveness of an injury prevention strategy in 2 groups of athletes—intervention and control—and both have the same number of injuries, it could prematurely be concluded that there was no preventative effect in the intervention group. What if,

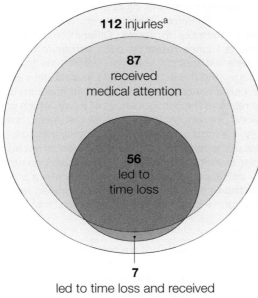

112 injuries[a]

87
received
medical attention

56
led to
time loss

7
led to time loss and received
no medical attention

Fig. 2. Number of injuries registered in a 1-season cohort of elite field hockey players. Reference: https://doi.org/10.1111/sms.13065. This example shows how different injury definitions (ie, all athlete self-reported injuries, injuries receiving medical attention, and injuries leading to training/match time loss) have an impact on the observed magnitude of the injury problem within a study. [a] An injury was defined as disorders of the musculoskeletal system or concussion. (*Adapted from* Clarsen B, Bahr R. Matching the choice of injury/illness definition to study setting, purpose and design: one size does not fit all! Br J Sports Med 2014;48(7):510–2; with permission.)

however, the athletes in the intervention group had played 5000 hours and those in the control group only 2500? The intervention group would have been more exposed to the risk of sustaining a sport injury than the control group and yet had the same number of injuries.

Combining the number of injuries with exposure data brings the concept of what is generally called injury rate.[22] Injury rates are usually described as the number of injuries per 1000 athlete-hours, which is calculated by dividing the total number of injuries by the total number of athlete-hours multiplied by 1000. Injury rates can also be expressed by the number of injuries per 1000 athlete-exposures (ie, sessions), albeit hours is preferred to take into account potential differences in length of training and match sessions.[22] Following the previous example, if both groups had 30 injuries, the injury rates in the intervention and control groups would be 6 injuries and 12 injuries per 1000 athlete-hours of exposure, respectively. Although the numbers of injuries were the same in both groups, the injury rate in the intervention group was half compared with the control group. Therefore, measuring exposure data in sports injuries research is highly recommended to enable the reporting of injury rates.[22]

Severity of Injury

When it comes to prevention of sports injuries, reducing both the number and severity of injuries is an interest.[7] An injury prevention strategy could also be considered successful when reducing the severity of injuries, even without a reduction in the absolute number of injuries.[23] Therefore, injury severity is an important outcome when assessing preventative strategies in sports. Different measures of severity have been described in sports injuries research, such as nature of injury, recovery time (ie, injury duration), received medical attention, sport time loss, work/school time loss, permanent damage, and the economic cost to treat the injury.[24] The impact of an injury on athletes' performance is also an important measure of injury severity.[25]

Severity measures relate to the consequences of injury, which can be measured at various levels (described previously). These severity measures, however, are strongly correlated.[24] Arguably, the most commonly used severity measure of sports injuries is days of sport time loss. Although important, some injuries do not lead to time loss and, therefore, require other severity measures (eg, injury impact on athlete performance). Similarly to the injury definition, the severity measure within a study is based on the context of the surveillance and research question; however, uniform measures between studies would improve comparability of research data.[24]

Compliance and Adherence

The extent to which study participants uptake and use an intervention as prescribed is a critical yet often overlooked outcome measure in injury prevention studies.[26] Although the importance of compliance and adherence is evident, the way compliance is dealt with in preventative studies is subject to a large degree of heterogeneity.[27] Valid and reliable tools to measure and report compliance and adherence are needed and should be matched to uniform definitions of both constructs. In efficacy trials (eg, RCTs), intervention uptake is defined as compliance, referring to the act of a participant conforming to recommendations with regard to prescribed dosage, timing, and frequency of an intervention.[28] In effectiveness trials, intervention uptake is regarding adherence, which refers to a process influenced by the environment and recognizes that user behavior is determined by social contexts and personal lifestyle.[29]

There is substantial heterogeneity in the way that studies on sports injury prevention have defined, measured, and reported the extent to which participants actually uptake preventative interventions.[26] These measurements are often derived from a supervisor (eg, coach) or by the athletes in case of a nonsupervised intervention (eg, home-based exercises). This information can be collected via paper sheets or online reports and can also be supplemented with random (unannounced) visits or phone calls by investigators/researchers. Similar to the definition and severity of injuries, definitions and measurements of compliance and adherence are diverse, and uniformity would facilitate interpretation and comparison of studies on sports injuries prevention.[26]

COMMON STATISTICS IN INJURY PREVENTION STUDIES
Difference and Ratio of Injury Rates

As discussed previously, injury rate is usually described as the number of injuries per 1000 athlete-hours or athlete-exposures. A simplistic method to estimate the effect of an injury prevention strategy is to calculate the arithmetical difference or ratio between injury rates in an intervention and control group. The reasoning of a difference and a ratio calculation is that if there is no difference between groups, the results are 0 and 1, respectively. If the 95% confidence interval (CI) of the injury rate difference or injury rate ratio includes 0 or 1, respectively, it can be concluded there was no significant difference between groups.[30] The 95% CI states that the real difference or ratio lies somewhere inside the given range with a 95% certainty. For example, in **Table 1**, a rate ratio of an intervention and control group is 0.64. This point estimate

Table 1
Different statistical outcomes comparing the use of a structured exercise-based injury prevention program for children's soccer players (ie, "11+ kids" intervention group) and not using the program but the team's regular warm-up program (ie, control group)

	Intervention		Control		
Statistical Method	Number of Injuries	Injury Rate[a] (95% CI)	Number of Injuries	Injury Rate[a] (95% CI)	Outcome (95% CI)
RR	139	0.99 (0.84–1.17)	235	1.55 (1.36–1.76)	RR 0.64 (0.52–0.79)
RD	139	0.99 (0.84–1.17)	235	1.55 (1.36–1.76)	RD 0.56 (0.30–0.81)
Cox regression[b]	123	0.88 (0.74–1.05)	178	1.20 (1.03–1.38)	HR 0.59 (0.47–0.74)
Cox mixed effects[c]	139	0.99 (0.84–1.17)	235	1.55 (1.36–1.76)	HR 0.52 (0.32–0.86)

Abbreviations: HR, hazard ratio; RD, rate difference; RR, rate ratio.
[a] Number of injuries per 1000 athlete-hours of exposure to soccer.
[b] Adjusted for adjusted for age, age-independent body height, and match-training ratio.
[c] Adjusted for adjusted for team clustering, age, age-independent body height, and match-training ratio and taking into account multiple injuries of players.
From Rössler R, Junge A, Bizzini M, et al. A multinational cluster randomised controlled trial to assess the efficacy of "11+ kids": a warm-up programme to prevent injuries in children's football. Sports Med 2017. https://doi.org/10.1007/s40279-017-0834-8; with permission.

indicates that the intervention group had a 36% lower injury rate. The corresponding 95% CI (0.52–0.79) shows that the observed intervention effect was statistically significant. Assume that the sample size of this study was not large enough to investigate the intervention effect with sufficient accuracy. Consequently, the observed point estimate of the rate ratio could still be the same (ie, 0.64) but due to the smaller sample size the 95% CI would be wider and might include 1 (eg, 0.30–1.20). In this scenario, firm conclusions cannot be drawn on the efficacy of the intervention due to the non-statistically significant effect.

Cox Regression Analysis

The Cox regression analysis has advantage over the injury rate difference or ratio because it takes into account an athlete's individual time at risk of sustaining an injury (ie, athlete-specific sport exposure data) and not only the summarized injury rate of a group. The outcome of a Cox regression analysis is the hazard ratio, which is a combination of 2 measures—the difference in proportion of injured athletes in the intervention and control group and the difference in the time to injury (ie, sport exposure data) between groups. In addition, a Cox regression analysis permits adjustment for confounders and the investigation of potential effect modifiers.[31] An example of a Cox regression analysis to assess the efficacy of a preventative strategy is shown in **Table 1**. In this example, the hazard ratio was 0.59, which means that the risk of sustaining an injury in the intervention group was 41% lower compared with the control group. A limitation of the original Cox regression analysis, however, is that it is only able to handle the first injury sustained by an athlete, ignoring all potential exposure and subsequent injury data after the first injury.[31] Furthermore, it cannot handle clustered data (eg, players nested in teams).

Cox Regression with Subsequent Events and/or Clustered Data

The limitations of the original Cox regression analysis, discussed previously, are important because athletes might sustain multiple injuries during a study. Extensions of the Cox regression analysis allow analyzing more than 1 injury of individual athletes.

Additionally, these extended Cox models take into account that subjects who sustained an injury are probably at a higher risk to sustain another injury. Furthermore, it is possible to account for a hierarchical data structure—for example, multiple injuries in an athlete, athletes nested in teams, and teams nested in clubs.[31] For these reasons, extended Cox models can be seen as more realistic than the traditional Cox regression analysis.[32] In the example in **Table 1**, the hazard ratio of an extended Cox regression was 0.52. Because this extended Cox model considered what happened with athletes after their first injury, in contrast with the original Cox regression, it can be concluded that at any point in time, the risk of sustaining an injury in the intervention group was 48% lower than in the control group.

Considering Adherence in the Analysis

The examples provided have illustrated comparison between 2 groups—intervention (ie, using a preventative strategy under investigation) and control. Analyzing outcomes according to participants' original group allocation characterizes an intention-to-treat analysis. This approach dismisses any potential deviations from the intervention protocol.[33] In real-life situations, however, protocols often do not happen exactly as planned a priori. This is also the case in preventative strategies for sports injuries, where participants' compliance and adherence to the intervention may deviate from the original plan.

Studies that accounted for compliance and adherence to preventative strategies demonstrated that they significantly affect outcomes.[26] Naturally, preventative strategies do not work if they are not used. This is illustrated by Verhagen and colleagues,[34] who showed a strong dose-response relationship between adherence to a prescribed training program and intervention effects (**Table 2**). As shown in this study, and which most likely is also the case in other preventative measures, the actual effects found are due to a relatively small subpopulation who adhered sufficiently to the prescribed intervention. The actual preventative effect in the intervention is, as such, greater than shown in the outcomes that are derived in an intention-to-treat analysis.

Table 2
Number of incident ankle sprain recurrences and ankle sprain recurrence incidence densities (95% CI) for various adherence categories

	Participants (% of Total)	Ankle Sprain Recurrences	Injury Rate (ie, Number of Injuries per 1000 Participant-Hours of Exposure)
Intervention group[a]	256	56	1.86 (1.37–2.35)
Full adherence	58 (23)	4	0.52 (0.01–1.04)
Partial adherence	75 (29)	21	2.02 (1.16–2.89)
No adherence	89 (35)	30	3.04 (1.95–4.13)
Control group	266	89	2.90 (2.30–3.50)

[a] Participants rated a 5-point scale twice during the study: "I performed the exercises of the program as prescribed." Participants rating 4 or 5 twice were considered fully adherent. Participants who scored a 4 or a 5 in only 1 of the 2 occasions were termed partially adherent. Participants who gave scores of 3 or lower on both occasions were considered not to have adhered to the prescribed intervention.
Adapted from Verhagen EALM, Hupperets MDW, Finch CF, et al. The impact of adherence on sports injury prevention effect estimates in randomised controlled trials: looking beyond the CONSORT statement. J Sci Med Sport 2011;14(4):289; with permission.

Considering Severity Measures in the Analysis

Injury burden on athletes' sport participation

As discussed previously, injury prevention studies are interested in reducing the rate and severity of injuries.[7] These 2 outcomes are usually reported separately, such as number of injuries per 1000 athlete-hours and days of sport time loss due to injury. It also possible, however, to account for both constructs in 1 measure and describe the cumulative days of time loss per 1000 athlete-hours. This measure is a cross-product of injury rate and severity—in this case days of sport time loss—and is referred to in sports medicine literature as injury burden.[35–37] **Fig. 3** illustrates, based on original data from a trial on a preventative warm-up intervention in youth field hockey, the value of taking injury burden into account in the analyses. If burden would not have been taken into account, it would have been concluded, based on the descriptive statistics, that the intervention did not lead to a significant reduction in injury rates, given the overlap of the confidence intervals of the intervention and control group. The injury burden was significantly lower, however, in the intervention group. Alternatively, the difference or ratio between the intervention and control group in regard to the injury burden can be calculated following the same reasoning of the difference or ratio of injury rates, described previously. By calculating the difference in **Fig. 3** example, it can be concluded that the intervention group had 8.42 (95% CI, 4.37–12.47) fewer days of sport time loss per 1000 athlete-hours.

Economic evaluations

A cost-effectiveness analysis is 1 form of economic evaluations that determines the efficiency of an intervention by comparing the costs and effects of 2 or more interventions.[38] Because cost data are positively skewed—most athletes have no injury and no costs and most injuries lead to minimal costs—nonparametric bootstrapping is considered the most appropriate method to analyze differences in costs. The outcomes of bootstrapped cost and effectiveness comparisons can then be graphically depicted in a so-called cost-effectiveness plane. For each intervention, the effect is plotted against the costs of the intervention and compared to a control group

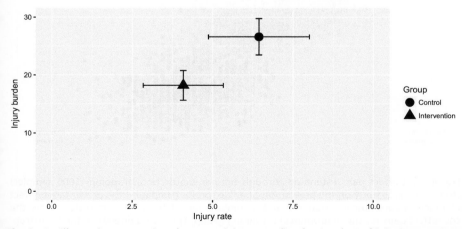

Fig. 3. An illustrative comparison between injury rate (ie, the number of injuries per 1000 player-hours of exposure to sport) and injury burden (ie, the number of sessions lost due to injury per 1000 player-hours of exposure to sport) when assessing the effectiveness of a preventative strategy in youth field hockey.

(eg, usual care). The cost-effectiveness plane provides an illustration of the relationship between competing interventions or intervention versus controlled condition in a scatter plot. **Fig. 4** presents such a plane from a previous study comparing the preventative effect of braces, neuromuscular training, and a combination of both on ankle sprains recurrences.[39] This plane shows that a brace is more cost-effective (ie, more effective and with lower costs) compared with neuromuscular training or a combination of bracing and neuromuscular training.

The so-called incremental cost-effectiveness ratio (ICER) describes how much additional benefit and at what additional cost an intervention program provides. The ICER is calculated by dividing the net costs of the program minus the net costs of standard care divided by the effectiveness of the program minus the effectiveness of the standard care. Typically, the ICER is given by units of currency per effectiveness gained.[40] For the example in **Fig. 4**, the ICER was 2828. This means that preventing 1 ankle sprain recurrence in the brace group was associated with €2828 ($ 3495) cost savings in comparison to the combination group.

Care should be taken when interpreting such results because, in a cost-effectiveness analysis, the comparator should always be usual care treatment. When it concerns prevention, the usual care treatment may be no preventative intervention. This could be regarded as a full control group. This, however, is not always the case. The comparator group in the example in **Fig. 4**, for instance, was also provided

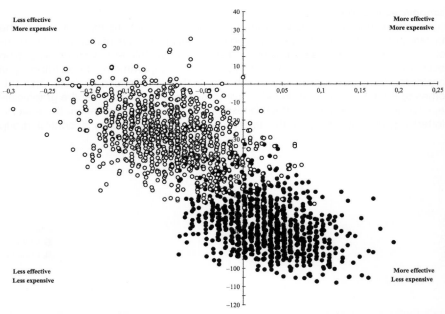

Fig. 4. Cost-effect pairs estimated through nonparametric bootstrapping (1000 samples) from a previous study on the prevention of ankle sprains comparing the preventative effect of braces, neuromuscular training, and a combination of both. The open dots show the cost-effect pairs for the neuromuscular training group. The closed dots show the bootstrapped cost-effect pairs for the brace group. Both groups are compared with the control group, who received a combination of both interventions. (*Data from* Janssen KW, Hendriks MRC, van Mechelen W, et al. The cost-effectiveness of measures to prevent recurrent ankle sprains: results of a 3-arm randomized controlled trial. Am J Sports Med 2014;42(7):1534–41.)

an effective preventative intervention, that is, neuromuscular training combined with bracing, as advised in the Dutch ankle sprain guidelines.[41] A cost-effectiveness analysis and the resulting ICER are to be interpreted only in relation to this comparator and as such may say nothing about the actual preventative and cost benefit of an intervention as a stand-alone preventative measure.

SUMMARY

This article provides a summary of the study designs, outcome measures, and common types of data analysis of sports injury prevention studies. There is no strict principle that should always be followed to ensure success in sports injury prevention research. Clinicians can use the information provided in this article to consider research findings and their context before applying preventative measures in practice.

REFERENCES

1. Lee I-M, Shiroma EJ, Lobelo F, et al. Effect of physical inactivity on major noncommunicable diseases worldwide: an analysis of burden of disease and life expectancy. Lancet 2012;380(9838):219–29.
2. World Health Organization. Physical activity fact sheet. Available at: http://www.who.int/mediacentre/factsheets/fs385. Accessed November 7, 2017.
3. Warburton DER, Nicol CW, Bredin SSD. Health benefits of physical activity: the evidence. CMAJ 2006;174(6):801–9.
4. Verhagen E, Bolling C, Finch CF. Caution this drug may cause serious harm! Why we must report adverse effects of physical activity promotion. Br J Sports Med 2015;49(1):1–2.
5. Drew MK, Raysmith BP, Charlton PC. Injuries impair the chance of successful performance by sportspeople: a systematic review. Br J Sports Med 2017;51(16):1209–14.
6. Engebretsen L, Bahr R, Cook JL, et al. The IOC Centres of Excellence bring prevention to sports medicine. Br J Sports Med 2014;48(17):1270–5.
7. van Mechelen W, Hlobil H, Kemper HCG. Incidence, severity, aetiology and prevention of sports injuries. Sports Med 1992;14(2):82–99.
8. Loudon K, Treweek S, Sullivan F, et al. The PRECIS-2 tool: designing trials that are fit for purpose. BMJ 2015;350:h2147.
9. Singal AG, Higgins PDR, Waljee AK. A primer on effectiveness and efficacy trials. Clin Transl Gastroenterol 2014;5(1):e45.
10. Gartlehner G, Hansen RA, Nissman D, et al. Criteria for distinguishing effectiveness from efficacy trials in systematic reviews. Rockville (MD): Agency for Healthcare Research and Quality (US); 2006. Available at: http://www.ncbi.nlm.nih.gov/pubmed/20734508. Accessed November 30, 2017.
11. Sibbald B, Roland M. Understanding controlled trials: why are randomised controlled trials important? BMJ 1998;316(7126):201.
12. Rössler R, Junge A, Bizzini M, et al. A multinational cluster randomised controlled trial to assess the efficacy of "11+ kids": a warm-up programme to prevent injuries in children's football. Sports Med 2017. https://doi.org/10.1007/s40279-017-0834-8.
13. Rothwell PM. External validity of randomised controlled trials: "to whom do the results of this trial apply?". Lancet 2005;365(9453):82–93.
14. Vriend I, Gouttebarge V, Finch CF, et al. Intervention strategies used in sport injury prevention studies: a systematic review identifying studies applying the haddon matrix. Sports Med 2017;47(10):2027–43.

15. Sedgwick P. What is a non-randomised controlled trial? BMJ 2014;348:g4115.
16. Lincoln AE, Caswell SV, Almquist JL, et al. Effectiveness of the women's lacrosse protective eyewear mandate in the reduction of eye injuries. Am J Sports Med 2012;40(3):611–4.
17. Brown JC, Verhagen E, Knol D, et al. The effectiveness of the nationwide BokSmart rugby injury prevention program on catastrophic injury rates. Scand J Med Sci Sports 2016;26(2):221–5.
18. Benson BW. Head and neck injuries among ice hockey players wearing full face shields vs half face shields. JAMA 1999;282(24):2328.
19. Frieden TR. Evidence for health decision making — beyond randomized, controlled trials. N Engl J Med 2017;377(5):465–75.
20. Clarsen B, Bahr R. Matching the choice of injury/illness definition to study setting, purpose and design: one size does not fit all! Br J Sports Med 2014;48(7):510–2.
21. Mountjoy M, Junge A, Benjamen S, et al. Competing with injuries: injuries prior to and during the 15th FINA World Championships 2013 (aquatics). Br J Sports Med 2015;49(1):37–43.
22. de Loës M. Exposure data. Why are they needed? Sports Med 1997;24(3):172–5.
23. Rössler R, Donath L, Verhagen E, et al. Exercise-based injury prevention in child and adolescent sport: a systematic review and meta-analysis. Sports Med 2014; 44(12):1733–48.
24. van Mechelen W. The severity of sports injuries. Sports Med 1997;24(3):176–80.
25. Clarsen B, Rønsen O, Myklebust G, et al. The Oslo Sports Trauma Research Center questionnaire on health problems: a new approach to prospective monitoring of illness and injury in elite athletes. Br J Sports Med 2014;48(9):754–60.
26. van Reijen M, Vriend I, van Mechelen W, et al. Compliance with sport injury prevention interventions in randomised controlled trials: a systematic review. Sports Med 2016;46(8):1125–39.
27. McKay CD, Verhagen E. "Compliance" versus "adherence" in sport injury prevention: why definition matters. Br J Sports Med 2016;50(7):382–3.
28. Aronson JK. Compliance, concordance, adherence. Br J Clin Pharmacol 2007; 63(4):383–4.
29. Osterberg L, Blaschke T. Adherence to medication. N Engl J Med 2005;353(5): 487–97.
30. Hayen A, Finch CF. Statistics used in effect studies. In: Verhagen E, van Mechelen W, editors. Sports injury research. New York: Oxford University Press; 2009. p. 183–96.
31. Twisk J. Basic statistical methods. In: Verhagen E, van Mechelen W, editors. Sports injury research. New York: Oxford University Press; 2009. p. 19–40.
32. Ullah S, Gabbett TJ, Finch CF. Statistical modelling for recurrent events: an application to sports injuries. Br J Sports Med 2014;48(17):1287–93.
33. Sedgwick P. What is intention to treat analysis? BMJ 2013;346:f3662.
34. Verhagen EALM, Hupperets MDW, Finch CF, et al. The impact of adherence on sports injury prevention effect estimates in randomised controlled trials: looking beyond the CONSORT statement. J Sci Med Sport 2011;14(4):287–92.
35. Quarrie KL, Hopkins WG. Tackle injuries in professional rugby union. Am J Sports Med 2008;36(9):1705–16.
36. Fuller CW. Managing the risk of injury in sport. Clin J Sport Med 2007;17(3): 182–7.
37. Bahr R, Clarsen B, Ekstrand J. Why we should focus on the burden of injuries and illnesses, not just their incidence. Br J Sports Med 2017. https://doi.org/10.1136/bjsports-2017-098160.

38. Bosmans J, Heymans M, Hupperets M, et al. Cost-effectiveness studies. In: Verhagen E, van Mechelen W, editors. Sports injury research. New York: Oxford University Press; 2009. p. 197–212. https://doi.org/10.1093/acprof:oso/9780199561629.003.015.
39. Janssen KW, Hendriks MRC, van Mechelen W, et al. The cost-effectiveness of measures to prevent recurrent ankle sprains: results of a 3-arm randomized controlled trial. Am J Sports Med 2014;42(7):1534–41.
40. Cohen DJ, Reynolds MR. Interpreting the results of cost-effectiveness studies. J Am Coll Cardiol 2008;52(25):2119–26.
41. Kerkhoffs GM, van den Bekerom M, Elders LAM, et al. Diagnosis, treatment and prevention of ankle sprains: an evidence-based clinical guideline. Br J Sports Med 2012;46(12):854–60.

Considerations for Assessment and Applicability of Studies of Intervention

Alexandra B. Gil, PT, PhD*, Sara R. Piva, PT, PhD,
James J. Irrgang, PT, PhD

KEYWORDS

- Evidence-based practice • Hierarchy of evidence • Quality of evidence
- Applicability of evidence • Evidence-based medicine • Levels of evidence

KEY POINTS

- There are different study designs to test the benefits or harm of an intervention. Randomized clinical trials and systematic reviews are the strongest designs to minimize threats to validity.
- Quality indicators that impact the validity of intervention studies are sample representativeness, randomization, blinding, completeness of follow-up, data presentation, and chronology of data collection.
- The continuum between efficacy and effectiveness studies helps to determine the applicability of the evidence to individual patients.
- Efficacy studies are well-controlled and determine whether the intervention works under ideal circumstances; thus, treatment effects are greater than expected in clinical practice.
- Effectiveness studies sacrifice control to answer whether the intervention works under real clinical conditions and their treatment effects are similar to those expected in clinical practice.

INTRODUCTION

When evidence-based medicine emerged as a new approach to teach medical practice, the challenge to clinicians was clear: "Evidence-based medicine requires new skills of the physician, including efficient literature searching and the application of formal rules of evidence to evaluate the clinical literature."[1] Since then, the

Disclosure Statement: The authors have nothing to disclose.
Department of Physical Therapy, University of Pittsburgh, Bridgeside Point 1, 100 Technology Drive, Suite 210, Pittsburgh, PA 15219-3130, USA
* Corresponding author.
E-mail address: agil@pitt.edu

evidence-based medicine approach has crossed beyond the borders of medicine and, as Guyatt and colleagues[2] stated, this approach "applies to all clinical care provisions and the rubric evidence-based health care is equally appropriate." Despite all the good intentions of teaching the evidence-based practice approach to health care professionals, many clinicians do not have the necessary knowledge to evaluate the validity and usefulness of the medical literature.[3] The barriers experienced in the United States to implement evidence-based practice[4] are the same experienced in many other countries[5,6] and across the spectrum of health professions including sports medicine, physical therapy, and athletic training, just to mention a few.[4,7–9]

Several narratives have been published[10–13] with the intent to guide users of the evidence (ie, health care practitioners) on how to appraise the results of clinical research and apply to individual patients in everyday clinical practice. The goal of this review is to refresh clinicians' knowledge of the most important considerations while appraising the evidence of studies of intervention. This article first reviews the hierarchy of evidence and discuss the strengths and weaknesses of different study designs. Then, it discusses the elements of clinical studies that impact their validity followed by a description of the balance between internal and external validity. We hope this review helps clinicians, whatever their areas of practice, to feel empowered to be more active participants in the process of critically appraising and applying evidence to improve patient outcomes in their clinical practice.

HIERARCHY OF EVIDENCE FOR INTERVENTION STUDIES

The basis for clinical decision making relies on the interaction of evidence from clinically relevant research, clinical expertise, and patients' values. Health care practitioners must have the skills to distinguish high-quality from low-quality clinical research. To that end, hierarchies of evidence were developed to facilitate the work of busy clinicians in ranking research studies based on their study design and ability to minimize bias (ie, any tendency that prevents unprejudiced consideration of a question).[14] Hierarchies (or levels) of evidence are grades of recommendations for classifying studies based on research design, using internal validity as criterion for the rankings. Levels of evidence provide a short cut to finding the best evidence. For example, suppose a clinician wants to find evidence for exercise programs to prevent knee ligament injuries, but a search on the topic yields dozens of hits. The clinician then uses the levels of evidence to guide as to which articles are the most valid and useful for the purpose, and focuses first on systematic reviews (SRs). If those are not available, he goes down in the hierarchy and looks for randomized clinical trials (RCTs), and so on. Herein we present a summary of a hierarchy of evidence for intervention studies.[15] This hierarchy includes 5 levels, the lowest being mechanism-based reasoning studies and the highest being SRs of RCTs, which will be described from the bottom to the top level (**Fig. 1**).

Level V

Mechanistic studies establish the pathophysiologic basis for treatment and may be used to generate hypotheses or rule out implausible hypotheses and may provide preliminary evidence to support treatment efficacy in the absence of higher levels of evidence.[16] However, there is controversy regarding using mechanistic studies as a form of evidence to guide clinical practice.[15,16] Considering the purpose of this review, mechanistic studies are not discussed further.

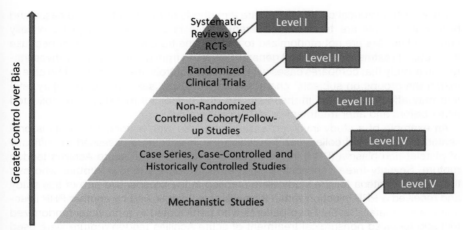

Fig. 1. Hierarchy of evidence for intervention studies. RCTs, randomized clinical trials.

Level IV

Case series involves a group or series of cases involving patients who were given similar treatment. They provide a description of a condition and outcomes for those patients. In this type of report, there is no control group for comparison, and outcomes measures are collected either before and after the intervention or after the intervention only.

The benefits of case series reside on the detailed description of a condition and the interventions being used (eg, the surgical procedure and/or rehabilitation program are generally described with sufficient detail to allow reliable replication). Additionally, case series contribute to the development of hypotheses that can be tested further with more rigorous study designs.[17] The main weakness in this type of report is the lack of a control group for comparison, which hinders the determination of whether changes in outcome measures are due to the intervention or another factor. For example, for self-limiting diseases, and improvements in pain and physical function observed after intervention could be simply the natural history of the condition. Additional threats to validity in case series are the potential for selection and information biases. Selection bias is common because the sample of these studies tends to be small and not represent consecutive patients who are treated for the condition nor are they randomly selected from the full spectrum of those with the disease. Information bias is common because the data are generally collected retrospectively from medical records, which have been traditionally incomplete and lack accuracy.

An example of a case series is an article published by McAleer and colleagues[18] in which 5 elite soccer players with confirmed pubic symphysis pain were treated with a nonoperative rehabilitation program. Each stage of the rehabilitation was reported in detail, including a clinical follow-up at least 8 months after return to play. All 5 players had reduced pain, increased strength of the adductor muscles, returned to pain-free soccer practice on average 41 days after treatment, and returned to playing soccer on average 49 days after treatment. The authors concluded that the nonoperative protocol may help patients affected by pubic symphysis pain to return to sports.[18] However, this study is limited by the small sample and lack of control group; so, one cannot infer that the treatment effect is due to the intervention versus the natural history of the condition.

Cases with historical controls compare 2 methods of treatment, but the cases and historical controls are treated at different points in time. Subjects in historically controlled studies are not randomized to receive one treatment or the other because the groups (treatment and control) generally originate from different studies. Investigators, in a study that compares cases with historical controls, may or may not be able to match the groups on subjects' characteristics (eg, age, sex, preexisting injury, etc) that may affect outcomes. In these studies, the outcomes measures are collected either before and after treatment or after treatment only.

An example of a study involving cases compared with historical controls is presented by Kaniki and colleagues[19] in which the investigators assessed the efficacy of platelet-rich plasma (PRP) in the nonsurgical treatment of acute Achilles tendon rupture. Seventy-three consecutive patients with Achilles tendon rupture who met the eligibility criteria for the study were enrolled in the prospective arm of this study and received a PRP injection within 2 weeks of injury followed by another PRP injection 2 weeks later. Seventy-two patients who participated in a previous randomized trial and received nonsurgical treatment of acute Achilles tendon rupture were used as a historical controls. The results indicated that PRP did not provide additive clinical benefit to the nonsurgical treatment.[19] Similar to case series, historically controlled studies are prone to information and selection biases. Although these studies have the benefit of a control group, a major disadvantage is that the lack of randomization may result in groups not being well-balanced in individuals' characteristics, and that may affect the study results.

Cases with concurrent controls (ie, case-control studies) are retrospective in nature (ie, the study is conceived after the data have been collected). The selection of cases is based on the presence of the outcome of interest and the selection of controls is based on the absence of the outcome of interest. This type of study looks back in time to determine if cases and controls differ on the exposure to factors that influence outcome, such as differences in treatment, personal characteristics, or risk factors. This design enables matching subjects on key characteristics that are known to contribute to outcome (eg, age, sex, body mass index, etc).

An example of a case-control study is one conducted by Danielsson and colleagues[20] in which their primary goal was to determine the long-term spinal mobility and muscle endurance of consecutive patients with adolescent idiopathic scoliosis treated with brace or surgery, and followed for at least 20 years. Two hundred thirty-seven patients treated with either procedure were identified using an existing registry, and 100 people matched by age and sex were selected to serve as the control group; none of these controls had spinal problems. The study results indicated that both treatment groups (brace and surgery) had less spinal mobility and muscle endurance compared with the control group (no scoliosis).[20]

Advantages of case-control studies are that the samples are easy to identify and these studies are useful for rare conditions or those with a long latency between the exposure and outcome. The inherent disadvantages of case-control studies include bias in the selection of the cases and controls, because it is generally not feasible to match groups on every factor related to disease or outcome, and consequent uncertainty about the relationship between the exposure and outcome despite having a control group.

Level III

Nonrandomized controlled prospective cohort studies compare 2 or more groups that receive different interventions, but the interventions are not randomly assigned to participants. These studies are planned before the enrollment of subjects and data on outcome measures are generally collected before and after the intervention. These may be the design of choice when funding is limited (randomized studies are very expensive) or to compare ongoing competing treatments from predetermined fixed groups, such as patients treated in a specialty clinic or students from a school (ie, when interventions are already being implemented on a large scale). This methodology is also an option when randomization is unethical. For example, for legal reasons, researchers cannot randomize athletes to take or not performance-enhancing drugs to determine the health-related side effects of those drugs, such as aggressiveness or mood changes. The disadvantage of these studies is that the lack of randomization may result in groups not similar in factors that may influence the study results. Many of these factors may not be subjected to analytical adjustments because investigators may not be aware of their existence and/or effect; thus, one cannot know if differences in outcomes between groups are due the group unbalances versus the intervention.

An example of a prospective nonrandomized controlled cohort is a study undertaken by Sillanpaa and colleagues[21] that compared the long-term outcomes of patients who suffered patellar dislocation treated with either acute arthroscopic stabilization or nonoperatively. They examined the number of redislocations, patient-reported symptoms, and level of physical function 7 years after the intervention. Investigators found that the rate of patellar redislocations were similar in both groups. Patients who underwent arthroscopic stabilization regained preinjury level of activity more often than those who did not undergo surgery.[21]

Level II

RCTs are prospective studies where subjects are randomly assigned to one treatment or another. The hallmark of this design is the random assignment of subjects, where every subject has the same chance to be assigned to each treatment arm. The theoretic assumption is that the randomization will similarly distribute subjects' characteristics across groups (the ones known and unknown to affect study outcome) and, therefore, isolate the effects of the experimental treatment. However, particularly in studies with small samples, there is a possibility that randomization will not be successful in creating similar groups, which needs to be assessed and clearly displayed in these studies.

In a study conducted by Kukkonen and colleagues,[22] 180 individuals with shoulder rotator cuff tear were randomized into 3 groups: (1) physical therapy only, (2) acromioplasty and physical therapy, or (3) rotator cuff repair, acromioplasty, and physical therapy. A nurse, unaware of treatment allocation, was responsible for randomization using a computer-generated sequence of numbers. Subjects' baseline characteristics (before interventions) displayed in a table demonstrated a similar distribution across groups. The results indicated no significant difference in clinical outcomes (ie, physical function, pain, and patient satisfaction) between the groups.

Level I

SRs of RCTs are a judicious synthesis of the results of carefully designed RCTs.[14,23] These reviews depend largely on the availability and quality of RCTs. However, in topics where there are no RCTs, SRs of cohort studies or case-control studies are appropriate, but these should not be considered a level 1 study to support the use of an intervention. When a sufficient number of studies that used similar outcome measures are available, the data on treatment effects from all studies may be pooled together using a process called metaanalysis. The analytics of metaanalyses involve calculation of odds ratios or relative risks for dichotomous data, and standardized mean differences for continuous data. Additionally, individual studies' sample size and variability have a direct impact on the pooled results of the metaanalysis. An example of an SR with metaanalysis is a study by Hughes and colleagues,[24] who systematically analyzed the literature to determine the effectiveness of blood flow restriction to the muscles in clinical musculoskeletal rehabilitation. A thorough search of RCTs in relevant databases was conducted. Two independent reviewers selected the studies, performed data extraction, and assessed the quality of individual studies. A metaanalysis was performed and its results indicated that low-load blood flow restriction is more effective and tolerable than low-load training and, thus, is a possible effective clinical rehabilitation tool.[24]

SRs with metaanalysis are foundational to evidence-based practice in guiding clinical decision making.[25] When well-conducted, they are powerful tools to draw conclusions related to treatment effectiveness from combined data from many smaller studies. However, if not well-conducted, just as any study discussed, the results of these syntheses may be misleading.[26]

QUALITY OF INTERVENTION STUDIES

Regardless of the ranking of a study within the hierarchy of the evidence, all forms of evidence, from level I to level V, should be appraised based on several quality indicators that may impact their validity. There are several useful tools to assess the quality of studies, depending on their design. For example, the PEDRO and JADAD scales are tools developed to assess the methodologic quality of clinical trials, whereas AMSTAR assesses the methodologic quality of SRs.[27–29] Furthermore, there are fundamental quality indicators that adversely impact the validity of studies and should always be considered, such as representativeness of the sample, randomization, blinding, duration and completeness of follow-up, data presentation, and timing of data collection. Common biases observed in clinical studies are discussed within the respective quality indicator that is most likely impacted by their presence (**Table 1**).

Representativeness of Sample

In clinical research, the population is the larger group of individuals with the condition of interest to which the research results are meant to be generalized.[17] For example, if a research study objective is to examine the effects of a treatment on people who had an Achilles tendon rupture, the population of interest would be composed of all individuals who have suffered an Achilles tendon rupture. However, because one cannot recruit all individuals with an Achilles tendon rupture, the sample is the portion of the population included in the study.[17] Sampling in clinical research generally involves selecting participants using nonrandom methods, such as convenience sampling, resulting in research volunteers who might be different on certain variables than nonvolunteers, which might make it difficult to generalize the results to the entire population.

The study eligibility criteria help to define whether the results obtained from the study sample may be generalized to the target population. The use of broad (few) inclusion criteria promotes external validity by enrolling individuals with the condition of interest who are similar to those who would be candidates to receive the intervention being tested. Conversely, with the use of restrictive (several) exclusion criteria, the similarities between the sample and the target population tend to decrease, thus reducing external validity.[30] For example, purposely excluding individuals less likely to respond to an intervention (those who may not adhere to the intervention or are not expected to remain in the study for its entirety) undermine the generalizability of

Table 1
Common biases in clinical studies, its definitions, and how to minimize them

Type	Definition	How to Minimize It
Sampling bias	Individuals in the sample either over or underrepresent population characteristics	Use of random selection of research participants Use of minimal inclusion/exclusion criteria Larger study samples
Selection bias	Systematic differences between baseline characteristics of the groups that are compared	Use of random allocation through a table of random sequenced numbers and adequate allocation concealment
Participant bias	Participant is aware of treatment assignment and changes behavior as a function of it	Blinding of research participant
Assessor bias	A tendency by the assessor to see what he or she expects to see, or want to see because of knowledge of subject treatment assignment	Blinding of outcomes assessor
Attrition bias	Systematic difference between groups in withdrawals from a study	Adjustment of target sample size to account for expected attrition Use of intention-to-treat analysis Use worst-case scenario to assess the results
Recall bias	Systematic error owing to an inability to retrieve complete or accurate data by memory	Use high-quality questionnaires, highly trained interviewers, and strategies to trigger memory Use prospective study design

a study. Last, sample size is also a consideration for sample representativeness. In general, the larger the study sample, the smaller the difference between characteristics in the population and the sample[31]; thus, the results of large studies tend to be more generalizable.

Randomization

Random allocation of subjects to intervention groups is a hallmark of RCTs. As discussed, it creates balanced groups and increases one's confidence that the study results are due to the intervention instead of differences between groups on potential unbalanced prognostic variables.[17,29] All study designs discussed, except for RCTs and SRs of RCTs, fail in respect to this indicator of high quality. Therefore, when assessing the validity of intervention studies, one should check the randomization process, including whether the random sequence was generated by an independent person using appropriate methods, such as a table of random sequenced numbers or computer-generated numbers. Moreover, to prevent selection bias, the person responsible for randomization (ie, revealing the number sequence and allocating participants into treatment groups) should not be involved with selecting participants into the study and the person selecting participants should not be involved with the allocation process, which is called allocation concealment. Allocation concealment prevents influencing which participants are assigned to a particular intervention group.

Different techniques can enhance the randomization process, such as the use of blocks, stratification, and covariate adaptive randomization.[32,33] Block randomization is when researchers divide participants into subgroups called blocks and then participants within each block are randomly assigned to treatment conditions.[34] Block randomization is generally not used in large studies where simple (complete) randomization is trusted to generate similar numbers of subjects across groups; however, in small studies, block randomization is helpful to balance the study groups. Stratified randomization is when subjects are first grouped based on strata (level) of a prognostic variable(s) that may affect outcome. Within each stratum, separate randomization schedules assign subjects to each treatment group.[35] Covariate adaptive randomization is done to balance groups on several important prognostic variables. With this method, a new subject is sequentially assigned to a treatment group by taking into account the specific covariates and previous assignments of participants.[36]

Randomization may be done at the level of the individual, which is the most common method, or cluster (group), of individuals.[37] Examples of clusters are medical practices randomized to administer or not an intervention to patients, and school districts randomized to provide or not injury prevention programs. Cluster randomization is preferred when the interventions are more naturally applied at the cluster level, for administrative convenience, or to protect against treatment contamination.[37] For example, Walden and colleagues[38] used soccer clubs as the unit of randomization (rather than individual subjects). They cluster randomized 230 Swedish clubs, from which 121 provided preventive neuromuscular training to adolescent female soccer players, and 109 did not. They reported a 64% decrease in the rate of anterior cruciate ligament injury in the intervention group compared with the control group.

Blinding

Blinding is expected to protect the study from bias if the behavior of the patient, clinician, or assessor may be influenced by knowledge of group assignment. Subjects may change their efforts toward achieving an outcome based on excitement or frustration related to knowing group assignment, and clinicians/assessors may involuntarily influence subjects' efforts toward achieving an outcome. Lack of blinding may influence the size of treatment effect. Therefore, whenever possible, clinical studies should blind patients, assessors, interventionists, investigators, and statisticians (ie, single-blinding, double-blinding, triple-blinding, and so forth).

In rehabilitation and orthopedic surgery, it is often difficult to blind both the subjects and the clinicians delivering the intervention, especially if one of the groups is a control group that receives no intervention. For example, in a study that offers surgery versus no surgery, both patients and surgeons cannot be blinded to group allocation.

Some studies have placed great efforts to blind subjects. One such study is that by Moseley and colleagues,[39] in which patients with knee osteoarthritis were randomized into 3 arms: (1) arthroscopic debridement, (2) arthroscopic lavage, or (3) placebo surgery. The subjects in the placebo group were prepped for an arthroscopic debridement procedure, including partial sedation, and received three 1-cm incisions that simulated the portals for the arthroscope.[39]

Blinding the assessor is usually easier, and should always be attempted. However, in small studies with limited funding/resources, that may not be feasible and the study team may have to rely on the clinician who delivered the intervention to also assess the outcomes. When blinding of the assessor is not possible, it is recommended to use outcome measures less influenced by assessor bias, such as patient-reported outcomes.

Completeness of Follow-up

Attrition refers to the loss of subjects (eg, withdrawal, drop-outs) along the course of the study. Like randomization and blinding, attrition may impact estimates of treatment effect in different ways.[17] Attrition can undermine successful randomization because, by the time the study is completed, the groups may no longer be balanced in key characteristics. Subjects who are lost to follow-up may also do so for various reasons, including treatment intolerance, loss of interest, or worsening of symptoms; thus, those who withdraw tend to have worse outcomes. Additionally, because attrition decreases the sample size, it may negatively impact the study's ability to identify differences between groups (ie, lower statistical power). Last, attrition may create a study sample no longer representative of the population of interest, thus compromising the generalizability of the results. A good rule of thumb is that a greater than 20% dropout rate poses a threat to the validity of the study results. However, it is important to note that a 20% dropout at a short-term follow up (eg, 6 weeks) is more of a concern than at a long-term follow-up (eg, 2 years) or if the dropouts mostly take place in one group versus another. In an attempt to minimize the impact of attrition, researchers may increase their target sample size to account for expected loss to follow-up.

Presentation of Data

Studies should describe baseline demographic and biomedical factors to enable comparison of key characteristics across groups and assessment of representativeness of the sample to the target population.[40] It is also important that studies report the results for each group with the estimated treatment effect (eg, mean changes or differences, odds ratios, or relative risks) and their precision (eg, confidence intervals, standard deviations) across all time points of data collection.[40] Furthermore, visual representation of data in graphs may help with the interpretation of results, such as box and whisker plots.[41] Without appropriate data presentation, readers are unable to assess both the clinical relevance of the results and the validity and impact of the study. For an in-depth discussion about analytics of clinical studies, please refer to the other articles within this issue.

Chronology of Data Collection

Intervention studies may be prospective or retrospective. Retrospective studies are more prone to bias because they use data that already exist (eg, medical records, health registries). These studies are initiated after the event of interest has occurred (eg, outcome after exposure to the intervention) and subjects are followed from the time point when the outcome occurred into the past and their exposure to treatment is recorded. Thus, subjects need to recollect events, which is often affected by memory bias, causing data to be incomplete or inaccurate. Conversely, in prospective studies the researchers follow subjects forward in time. Prospective studies are preferable because the data to be collected are determined before the study begins and the likelihood to obtain complete and accurate data is greater than for retrospective studies.

THE SPECTRUM OF EFFICACY AND EFFECTIVENESS STUDIES

Consumers of research evidence benefit from well-designed intervention studies, particularly RCTs. There are elements of the design of intervention studies (eg, recruitment strategy, study setting, method of intervention delivery, and selection of outcome measures) that should be assessed by consumers of evidence because they influence the placement of studies in the continuum of efficacy and effectiveness (**Fig. 2**) and dictate whether the results can be generalized to other situations and to other people.[30]

Efficacy (explanatory) studies (see **Fig. 2**, *left*) are designed to determine whether a treatment can work under a high level of control (internal validity) and ideal circumstances.[42] These studies serve as a proof of concept (pilot) to pave the way for larger effectiveness studies. They enroll selective subjects who are likely to adhere to and benefit from the intervention, and exclude those with conditions that may confound study results. Testing and intervention protocols are rigidly standardized and administered by highly trained personnel in laboratory setting to minimize variation. Both testers and participants and generally blinded. These usually include outcome measures of mechanisms by which the intervention work and do not include noncompliers in the analysis (per-protocol or as-treated analysis). These combined strategies avoid confounding and result in effect sizes that are generally greater than the ones observed in pragmatic trials; thus, efficacy studies require smaller sample size than the pragmatic ones. It is important to note that the treatment effects from efficacy studies tend to be greater than the ones expected in clinical practice because real patients do not behave as research participants (eg, most patients are not compliant and have coexisting conditions) and health care settings are not as ideal as in efficacy studies.

In contrast, effectiveness (pragmatic) studies (see **Fig. 2**, *right*) test whether patients benefit from treatment under usual (real-world) clinical circumstances and promote external validity/generalizability.[17,30] These studies enroll everyone with the condition of interest regardless of coexisting confounding conditions. Testing and intervention protocols are highly flexible and administered as usual in routine care. Clinicians and patients are generally not blinded. Outcome measures are important to participants and generally used in routine course of care. Analysis includes all participants who entered the trial regardless if they completed the study or not (intention-to-treat). Nonstrict control over these elements of study design result in more confounding and smaller treatment effects in pragmatic trials compared with efficacy studies. Consequently these studies require larger sample sizes to identify differences between study groups.

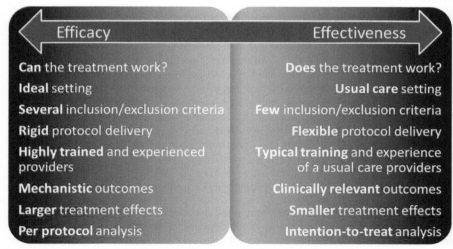

Fig. 2. Continuum of explanatory and programmatic studies.

Very few studies are purely explanatory or pragmatic. Most are compromises with mixed priorities and are placed within both extremes of this continuum and are exemplified next.[43] Piva and colleagues[44] conducted a single-center pilot randomized study to test whether balance exercises would be feasible/safe and promote physical function in patients greater than 2 months after total knee replacement. This study has features that place it closer to the efficacy end of the continuum. They randomized 43 individuals (small sample) to either functional training or functional training supplemented with a balance exercise program. The study created an ideal environment by controlling factors that could provide competing explanations for the effects of the intervention. For instance, only 1 experienced orthopedic surgeon was the source of recruitment; therefore, all subjects underwent the same surgical and inpatient rehabilitation procedures. Eligibility criteria were narrow to create a sample that was safe to exercise (eg, able to ambulate 100 ft without rest or the use of an assistive device) and likely to respond positively to the intervention (eg, excluded those with chronic conditions). The interventions were delivered in an academic setting by highly trained physical therapists who provided one-to-one attention to the participants. Testers were periodically trained in the research protocol. In addition, participant compliance was measured regularly. Last, only patients who completed the study were included in the analysis.[44] Under these highly controlled conditions, study participants who completed the study were more likely to have had greater treatment responses, which may not be generalizable to the general population.

Griffin and colleagues[45] conducted an effectiveness study with the goal to compare the benefits of open reduction with internal fixation surgery versus nonoperative treatment for displaced intraarticular calcaneal fractures. This study is closer to the effectiveness end of the continuum because the study methodology focused on maximizing the generalizability of the results. There were few inclusion/exclusion criteria; thus, the study sample closely resembled the population of interest. This multicenter study recruited participants from 22 hospitals, which were referral centers for calcaneal fractures and the surgeons were certified specialists in the repair of these injuries. The surgical technique used was standard of care at the UK and the postoperative care was managed by a standardized rehabilitation program. Furthermore, the outcome measures included pain, physical function, and quality of life, which are clinically relevant outcomes, readily available in the clinic, and did not require special training. Last, an intention-to-treat analysis was carried out.[45] Under such real-world conditions, the expectation is that the effects of the intervention are more realistic representations of the true treatment effect.

SUMMARY

In this article, we refreshed the clinicians' knowledge of important considerations while appraising the evidence of intervention studies. We hope that this information will help clinicians in interpreting the validity and results applicability of any clinical study. This skill is especially important in light of known contradictions and large effects of high profile studies that have been overturned after replication.[46,47] The lack of the knowledge to determine to what extent studies are truly valid, the extent to which the design elements impact estimates of the treatment effects, and where studies belong on the continuum of efficacy and effectiveness may delay or inadvertently affect advances in clinical practice. If readers are able to appraise the impact of these important study considerations, in addition to understanding strengths and weaknesses of study designs, they will have a more comprehensive understanding and ability to apply the clinical findings their patients, in their clinical environment. In this article, we have attempted to provide the reader with this information.

REFERENCES

1. Evidence-Based Medicine Working Group. Evidence-based medicine. A new approach to teaching the practice of medicine. JAMA 1992;268(17):2420–5.
2. Guyatt GH, Haynes RB, Jaeschke RZ, et al. Users' guides to the medical literature: XXV. Evidence-based medicine: principles for applying the users' guides to patient care. Evidence-Based Medicine Working Group. JAMA 2000;284(10): 1290–6.
3. Ioannidis JPA, Stuart ME, Brownlee S, et al. How to survive the medical misinformation mess. Eur J Clin Invest 2017;47(11):795–802.
4. Jette DU, Bacon K, Batty C, et al. Evidence-based practice: beliefs, attitudes, knowledge, and behaviors of physical therapists. Phys Ther 2003;83(9):786–805.
5. Ramirez-Velez R, Bagur-Calafat MC, Correa-Bautista JE, et al. Barriers against incorporating evidence-based practice in physical therapy in Colombia: current state and factors associated. BMC Med Educ 2015;15:220.
6. Chiu YW, Weng YH, Wahlqvist ML, et al. Do registered dietitians search for evidence-based information? A nationwide survey of regional hospitals in Taiwan. Asia Pac J Clin Nutr 2012;21(4):630–7.
7. Aarons GA, Wells RS, Zagursky K, et al. Implementing evidence-based practice in community mental health agencies: a multiple stakeholder analysis. Am J Public Health 2009;99(11):2087–95.
8. Welch CE, Hankemeier DA, Wyant AL, et al. Future directions of evidence-based practice in athletic training: perceived strategies to enhance the use of evidence-based practice. J Athl Train 2014;49(2):234–44.
9. Manspeaker S, Van Lunen B. Overcoming barriers to implementation of evidence-based practice concepts in athletic training education: perceptions of select educators. J Athl Train 2011;46(5):514–22.
10. Guyatt GH, Sackett DL, Cook DJ. Users' guides to the medical literature. II. How to use an article about therapy or prevention. A. Are the results of the study valid? Evidence-Based Medicine Working Group. JAMA 1993;270(21):2598–601.
11. Cleland JA, Noteboom JT, Whitman JM, et al. A primer on selected aspects of evidence-based practice relating to questions of treatment. Part 1: asking questions, finding evidence, and determining validity. J Orthop Sports Phys Ther 2008;38(8):476–84.
12. Noteboom JT, Allison SC, Cleland JA, et al. A primer on selected aspects of evidence-based practice to questions of treatment. Part 2: interpreting results, application to clinical practice, and self-evaluation. J Orthop Sports Phys Ther 2008;38(8):485–501.
13. Petticrew M, Roberts H. Evidence, hierarchies, and typologies: horses for courses. J Epidemiol Community Health 2003;57(7):527–9.
14. Jewell DV. Guide to evidence-based physical therapist practice. 4th edition. Burlington (MA): Jones & Bartlett Learning; 2018.
15. Howick J, Chalmers I, Glasziou P, et al. The 2011 Oxford CEBM levels of evidence (Introductory Document). Oxford Centre for Evidence-Based Medicine. Available at: https://www.cebm.net/index.aspx?o=5653. Accessed March 13, 2018.
16. Howick J, Glasziou P, Aronson JK. Evidence-based mechanistic reasoning. J R Soc Med 2010;103(11):433–41.

17. Portney LG, Watkins MP. Foundations of clinical research: applications to practice. Norwalk (CT): Appleton & Lange; 1993.

18. McAleer SS, Lippie E, Norman D, et al. Nonoperative management, rehabilitation, and functional and clinical progression of osteitis pubis/pubic bone stress in professional soccer players: a case series. J Orthop Sports Phys Ther 2017;47(9): 683–90.

19. Kaniki N, Willits K, Mohtadi NG, et al. A retrospective comparative study with historical control to determine the effectiveness of platelet-rich plasma as part of nonoperative treatment of acute Achilles tendon rupture. Arthroscopy 2014; 30(9):1139–45.

20. Danielsson AJ, Romberg K, Nachemson AL. Spinal range of motion, muscle endurance, and back pain and function at least 20 years after fusion or brace treatment for adolescent idiopathic scoliosis: a case-control study. Spine (Phila Pa 1976) 2006;31(3):275–83.

21. Sillanpaa PJ, Maenpaa HM, Mattila VM, et al. Arthroscopic surgery for primary traumatic patellar dislocation: a prospective, nonrandomized study comparing patients treated with and without acute arthroscopic stabilization with a median 7-year follow-up. Am J Sports Med 2008;36(12):2301–9.

22. Kukkonen J, Joukainen A, Lehtinen J, et al. Treatment of nontraumatic rotator cuff tears: a randomized controlled trial with two years of clinical and imaging follow-up. J Bone Joint Surg Am 2015;97(21):1729–37.

23. Higgins JPT, Green S. Cochrane handbook for systematic reviews of interventions version 5.1.0 [updated March 2011]. The Cochrane Collaboration 2011. Available at: www.handbook.cochrane.org. Accessed March 13, 2018.

24. Hughes L, Paton B, Rosenblatt B, et al. Blood flow restriction training in clinical musculoskeletal rehabilitation: a systematic review and meta-analysis. Br J Sports Med 2017;51(13):1003–11.

25. Bax L, Ikeda N, Fukui N, et al. More than numbers: the power of graphs in meta-analysis. Am J Epidemiol 2009;169(2):249–55.

26. Israel H, Richter RR. A guide to understanding meta-analysis. J Orthop Sports Phys Ther 2011;41(7):496–504.

27. Jadad AR, Moore RA, Carroll D, et al. Assessing the quality of reports of randomized clinical trials: is blinding necessary? Control Clin Trials 1996;17(1):1–12.

28. Shea BJ, Hamel C, Wells GA, et al. AMSTAR is a reliable and valid measurement tool to assess the methodological quality of systematic reviews. J Clin Epidemiol 2009;62(10):1013–20.

29. Physiotherapy Evidence Database (PEDro). Available at: https://www.pedro.org. au/. Accessed March 13, 2018.

30. Loudon K, Treweek S, Sullivan F, et al. The PRECIS-2 tool: designing trials that are fit for purpose. BMJ 2015;350:h2147.

31. Goodwin CJ. Research in psychology: methods and design. Hoboken (NJ): John Wiley and Sons; 2010.

32. Kim J, Shin W. How to do random allocation (randomization). Clin Orthop Surg 2014;6(1):103–9.

33. Kang M, Ragan BG, Park JH. Issues in outcomes research: an overview of randomization techniques for clinical trials. J Athl Train 2008;43(2):215–21.

34. Efird J. Blocked randomization with randomly selected block sizes. Int J Environ Res Public Health 2011;8(1):15–20.

35. Kernan WN, Viscoli CM, Makuch RW, et al. Stratified randomization for clinical trials. J Clin Epidemiol 1999;52(1):19–26.

36. Zhao W, Hill MD, Palesch Y. Minimal sufficient balance-a new strategy to balance baseline covariates and preserve randomness of treatment allocation. Stat Methods Med Res 2012;24(6):989–1002.
37. Hemming K, Eldridge S, Forbes G, et al. How to design efficient cluster randomised trials. BMJ 2017;358:j3064.
38. Walden M, Atroshi I, Magnusson H, et al. Prevention of acute knee injuries in adolescent female football players: cluster randomised controlled trial. BMJ 2012;344:e3042.
39. Moseley JB, O'Malley K, Petersen NJ, et al. A controlled trial of arthroscopic surgery for osteoarthritis of the knee. N Engl J Med 2002;347(2):81–8.
40. Moher D, Schulz KF, Altman DG, et al. The CONSORT statement: revised recommendations for improving the quality of reports of parallel-group randomized trials. Ann Intern Med 2001;134(8):657–62.
41. Weissgerber TL, Milic NM, Winham SJ, et al. Beyond bar and line graphs: time for a new data presentation paradigm. PLoS Biol 2015;13(4):e1002128.
42. Singal AG, Higgins PD, Waljee AK. A primer on effectiveness and efficacy trials. Clin Transl Gastroenterol 2014;5:e45.
43. Thorpe KE, Zwarenstein M, Oxman AD, et al. A pragmatic-explanatory continuum indicator summary (PRECIS): a tool to help trial designers. J Clin Epidemiol 2009; 62(5):464–75.
44. Piva SR, Gil AB, Almeida GJ, et al. A balance exercise program appears to improve function for patients with total knee arthroplasty: a randomized clinical trial. Phys Ther 2010;90(6):880–94.
45. Griffin D, Parsons N, Shaw E, et al. Operative versus non-operative treatment for closed, displaced, intra-articular fractures of the calcaneus: randomised controlled trial. BMJ 2014;349:g4483.
46. Ioannidis JP, Haidich AB, Pappa M, et al. Comparison of evidence of treatment effects in randomized and nonrandomized studies. JAMA 2001;286(7):821–30.
47. Ioannidis JP. Contradicted and initially stronger effects in highly cited clinical research. JAMA 2005;294(2):218–28.

A Picture Tells 1000 Words (but Most Results Graphs Do Not)

21 Alternatives to Simple Bar and Line Graphs

Jay Hertel, PhD, ATC[a,b,*]

KEYWORDS

- Data visualization • Graphs • Plots • Scientific writing

KEY POINTS

- Bar graphs and line graphs that plot group means and SDs do not provide readers with a thorough understanding of the distribution of individual participant measures.
- Investigators should consider alternatives to bar graphs and line graphs, such as dot plots or box and whisker plots, to visualize individual data points for studies with smaller sample sizes, and violin plots, to display full data distributions in studies with large sample sizes.
- Novel forms of graphs that can illustrate magnitudes of difference, strength of relationships, or multivariate relationships between measures should be considered when presenting research results.

INTRODUCTION

The adage, "a picture tells 1000 words," is often used by experienced investigators when mentoring students, residents, fellows, and other junior colleagues on the intricacies of scientific writing. Graphical representation of research results is often a more effective way to convey findings than text or tables. One wise scholar once told me the ultimate results section of an original research article should contain just 3 words: "see Figure 1." Alas, many investigators default to simple bar graphs or line graphs that are easy to make in common software packages but often have shortcomings when it comes to thoroughly illustrating research findings. When this happens, results figures may not be "worth 1000 words" and, more critically, they may not be a holistic visual representation of the study results.

Disclosure Statement: The author has no conflicts to disclose.
[a] Department of Kinesiology, University of Virginia, PO Box 400407, Charlottesville, VA 22904-4407, USA; [b] Department of Orthopaedic Surgery, University of Virginia, PO Box 800159, Charlottesville, VA 22908, USA
* Department of Kinesiology, University of Virginia, PO Box 400407, Charlottesville, VA 22904-4407.
E-mail address: Jhertel@virginia.edu

Clin Sports Med 37 (2018) 441–462
https://doi.org/10.1016/j.csm.2018.04.001
0278-5919/18/© 2018 Elsevier Inc. All rights reserved.
sportsmed.theclinics.com

The primary criticism of bar graphs and line graphs is that drastically different data sets can produce identical mean and SD (or SE) values. This phenomenon was first described by Anscombe[1] in 1973 and has more recently been championed in the life sciences by Weissgerber and colleagues.[2] The primary concern is that differences in group means may be driven by large differences from a small subset of research participants rather than by consistent differences across a majority of participants (**Fig. 1**). A related concern is that the depiction of data distribution with the group SD (or SE) may be a misleading representation of the distribution of a data set. These concerns have led to a call for investigators to explore alternative ways of illustrating research results with a particular emphasis on graphing the values obtained from individual participants in an effort to allow readers to fully comprehend relationships and trends in a data set.[2–11]

Another concern is that graphs of single, or a select handful of, outcome measures fail to describe the multifactorial relationships that often exist between variables.[7] Investigators frequently limit graphs to only 1 or 2 axes or dimensions, thus placing constraints on how data and relationships can be illustrated and interpreted. Advances in data visualization techniques should be used by investigators in an effort to best represent their research findings to readers. Clinicians and researchers are constantly combing the literature for novel developments in clinical and laboratory techniques; likewise, advances should be sought in methods to visualize research results.

The aim of this article is neither to provide a treatise on statistical distributions and analysis techniques nor to provide a tutorial on the step-by-step procedures of how to construct different types of graphs in specific software programs. Instead, the aim is to provide readers with a (nonexhaustive) set of alternatives to simple bar graphs and line graphs in an effort to spur thought and inspiration about the optimal way to illustrate results.

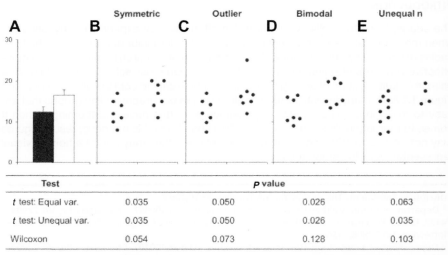

Test	p value			
t test: Equal var.	0.035	0.050	0.026	0.063
t test: Unequal var.	0.035	0.050	0.026	0.035
Wilcoxon	0.054	0.073	0.128	0.103

Fig. 1. Schematic of 4 data sets with nearly identical group means and SDs (*A*) but very different distributions (*B–E*). The dot plots provide readers with more information on trends in the data set than the bar graph. var, variances. (*From* Weissgerber TL, Milic NM, Winham SJ, et al. Beyond bar and line graphs: time for a new data presentation paradigm. PLoS Biol 2015;13(4):e1002128; with permission.)

ILLUSTRATING INDIVIDUAL PARTICIPANT MEASURES AND GROUP DISTRIBUTIONS
Univariate Scatterplot

Univariate scatterplots, also called dot plots, allow for each subject's measure of a single outcome to be illustrated (see **Fig. 1**B–E). The array of data for each group can be augmented with additional symbols for measures of central tendency, such as mean or median, and variability estimates, such as SD, SE, interquartile range, or CI. A univariate scatterplot can also be transposed on a traditional bar graph. The advantage of this type of graph is that it illustrates all data points and it is particularly useful for data sets with smaller sample sizes.[2]

Box and Whiskers Plot

An extension of the univariate scatter plot is the box and whiskers plot (**Fig. 2**), in which all subjects' data points are graphed vertically (parallel to the Y axis) and a box is formed so that the top and bottom depict the borders of the interquartile range (or other estimate of variability).[12] This box is typically intersected by a horizontal line representing the group median or, on some occasions, the mean. Often, whiskers extending from the top and bottom of the box plot extend to the maximum and minimum values in the data set. The advantage of the box and whiskers plot is that all data points are displayed along with a measure of central tendency and an estimate of variability. Data from different groups or time points can be shown on the same graph to allow for easy visual comparisons of the magnitude and dispersion. A limitation of box plot is that although the height of the box has tangible meaning (variability estimate) the width of the box does not.

Violin Plot

A violin plot builds on the limitation (discussed previously) of the box plot, namely ascribing meaning to both the height and width of the geometric figure that is graphed (**Fig. 3**). The length of the violin plot represents the range of measures in the data set extending from the minimum to the maximum scores, whereas the width represents

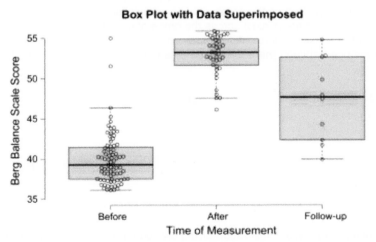

Fig. 2. Box plots provide visualization of the central tendency (median) and distribution (interquartile range and outliers) of a data set. (*From* Nuzzo RL. The box plots alternative for visualizing quantitative data. PM R 2016;8:269; with permission.)

the distribution of individual scores throughout the range. The widest point on a violin plot represents the mode. In the simplest sense, the right and left sides of the shape are mirror images of the histogram of the distribution of individual scores from the sample. Some investigators, however, choose to graph the probability density function rather than the actual sample distribution.[8] Additional encoding may be made within the graph to indicate values of central tendency and variability estimates. Violin plots are particularly useful for illustrating data sets that are large or have non-normal distributions. For example, a data set with a bimodal distribution is readily apparent in a violin plot but not in a box plot.

Graphing Individual Change Scores

Another extension of the univariate scatterplot for pre–post designs can be helpful for illustrating the change in measures for each individual subject between 2 time points[2] (**Fig. 4**). This type of graph can be useful for seeing whether all, or most, subjects had a consistent direction and magnitude of change or whether there is a subset of participants who demonstrated substantial changes (responders) and other subsets of participants who may have demonstrated minimal changes (nonresponders) or changes in the opposite direction. By plotting individual changes over time, this type of graphing does for the visualization of group mean differences what the univariate scatterplot does for group means.

Bland-Altman Plot

A Bland-Altman plot is a specific type of scatterplot that is used to visualize the results of studies comparing 2 measures[13,14] (**Fig. 5**). Specific cases could include the comparison of 2 testing devices or procedures to measure the same construct (eg, comparing maximal voluntary isometric contraction force measures using a handheld dynamometer vs an isokinetic dynamometer), comparison of 2 raters in an assessment of interrater reliability, or comparing repeated measures using the same measurement technique in a test-retest design. The X axis of a Bland-Altman plot represents the mean of the 2 measures taken for each participant, whereas the Y axis represents the arithmetical difference between the 2 measures. Each participant's scores are plotted on the graph yielding visualization of how similar the 2 measurement techniques are (Y axis) across the range of measurement values (X axis). In addition to the X axis, 3 horizontal lines are plotted: the middle line represents the mean difference between the 2 measurements (ideal value is 0) whereas the upper

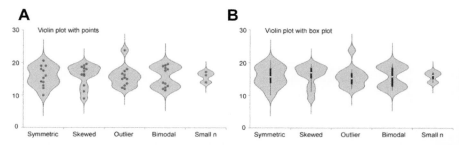

Fig. 3. Violin plots provide visualization of the distribution of a data set and can include presentation of individual data points (*A*) or components of a box and whiskers plot (*B*). (*From* Weissgerber TL, Savic M, Winham SJ, et al. Data visualization, bar naked: a free tool for creating interactive graphics. J Biol Chem 2017;292:20594; with permission.)

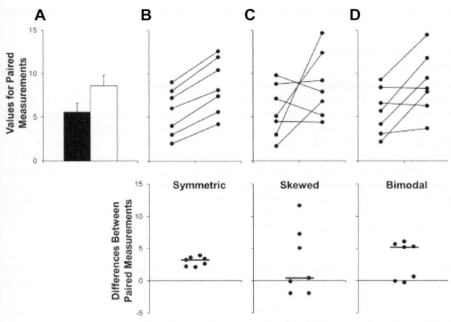

Fig. 4. Visualizing the pre–post change scores of each participant can provide readers with more information about the magnitude and direction of individual change scores than do group metrics. Note that pre–post group changes shown in the bar graph (*A*) could be due to very different pre–post changes in individual measures (*B–D*). (*From* Weissgerber TL, Milic NM, Winham SJ, et al. Beyond bar and line graphs: time for a new data presentation paradigm. PLoS Biol 2015;13(4):e1002128; with permission.)

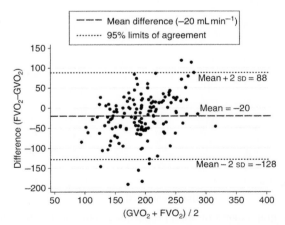

Fig. 5. Bland-Altman plot illustrating the relationship of 2 measurement techniques to assess oxygen consumption: inspired gas analysis (GVO_2) and the reverse Fick method (FVO_2) based on arterial and mixed venous blood gas analysis, respectively. The mean of each pair of measures is plotted on the X axis and the difference between each pair of measures is plotted on the Y axis. (*From* Myles PS, Cui J. Using the Bland–Altman method to measure agreement with repeated measures. Br J Anaesth 2007;99:310; with permission.)

and lower lines represent the 95% limits of agreement between the 2 measurement techniques.[13,14]

ILLUSTRATING PROPORTIONS
Stacked Bar Graph

Although bar graphs have limitations when it comes to illustrating group means and variability estimates, they are beneficial for illustrating frequencies of count data or proportions. Stacked bar graphs are particularly well suited for displaying proportion data when there are a small number of categories (fewer than 4 or 5) within the whole (**Fig. 6**). An example is expressing the proportion of subgroup members within an entire sample of study participants (eg, the proportion of freshmen, sophomores, juniors, and seniors within a school-based data set). Stacked bar graphs also can be used to express proportions of multiple measures quantified on a continuous scale (eg, the proportion of muscle volume for each of the 4 quadriceps muscles in making up the volume of the entire muscle group), although a limitation of this approach is that it is difficult to illustrate any variability estimates.

Donut Chart

A donut chart is essentially a stacked bar graph that has been converted to a circle where the circumference of the circle, rather than the height of the bar, represents 100% of the sample. The proportion of data in each category is presented in a corresponding portion of the circle's circumference (**Fig. 7**). A drawback of donut charts is that their usefulness is limited to displaying the results of a single set of measures; thus, they are not useful in showing comparisons across multiple time points.

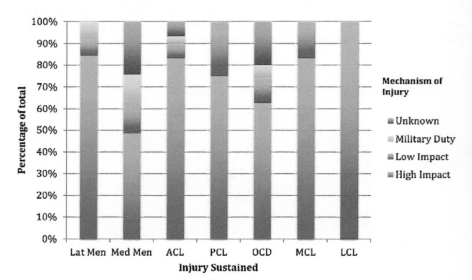

Fig. 6. Stacked bar graph demonstrating proportional data for the mechanism of different knee injuries according to confirmed injury on MRI. ACL, anterior cruciate ligament; Lat, lateral; LCL, lateral collateral ligament; MCL, medical colateral ligament; med, medial; men, meniscal; OCD, osteochondral defect; PCL, posterior cruciate ligament. (*From* Bell D, Wood A, Wrigley S, et al. Assessing the benefit of multidisciplinary assessment centre in a military population sustaining knee injury. J Arthroscopy Joint Surg 2015;2:109; with permission.)

Mosaic Plot

Illustration of the frequency in the outcomes of 2 or more categorical variables may be performed with a mosaic plot, also called a spineplot.[15] Mosaic plots are essentially a pictorial representation of a contingency table. Each combination of categories receives its own bin in which the area is proportional to the frequency of the total sample that lies within it (**Fig. 8**). Unlike bar graphs, where all bars are of the same width (but different height), the width and height of the different bins both can vary to represent smaller or larger proportions.

ILLUSTRATING MAGNITUDE OF DIFFERENCES AND RELATIONSHIPS
Forest Plot

Most often associated with meta-analyses, forest plots are effective at illustrating the magnitude of group differences identified across multiple comparisons. Each comparison represents a "tree," whereas the entire graph embodies the "forest" of related results. The X axis reflects a continuous scale representing the measure of magnitude that could be in the unit of measurement, such as group mean or group mean difference values, or on a unitless scale, such as effect size or odds ratio (**Fig. 9**). For each comparison reported, the point estimate and corresponding variability estimate, usually 95% CI, are plotted on the graph. The results of each comparison are displayed in series from top to bottom as the Y axis is not a numeric scale.

For meta-analyses, the size of the point estimate symbol is often manipulated to reflect the number of participants evaluated in a particular study with larger shapes equating to larger sample sizes. Another unique feature of a forest plot in the context of a meta-analysis is the graphing of the pooled estimate at the bottom of the series of scores (closest to the X axis). The pooled estimate is typically shown as a diamond whose height corresponds to the magnitude of the point estimate and width reflects the CI.

Heat Map

Reporting the results of a study that has a large number of dependent variables can be a challenge for even the most experienced author. Although presenting results in tables is an option, at a certain point the volume of tabular data can become unwieldy when dealing with numerous outcome measures. One approach to data visualization that has gained considerable popularity in recent years is the use of heat maps to illustrate the magnitude of results. In its simplest form, a heat map is a results table that replaces numbers with colors (**Fig. 10**). The spectrum of colors used corresponds to a scale of the numeric values represented. For example, blue, yellow, orange, and red could be operationally defined as representing trivial, small, moderate, and large effect sizes, respectively.

Heat maps are not limited to being color-coded tables. Everyone is likely familiar with weather maps that illustrate the expected temperatures in different geographic areas, where the ends of the temperature spectrum are red equating with hot temperatures and blue with cold temperatures. Similarly, in medical research, heat maps can be used to illustrate the magnitude of measures gathered from different anatomic regions (**Fig. 11**). Such visual representations of results are likely more intuitive to informed readers than sorting through myriad tabular results.

Speedometer Graph

Another means of visualizing the magnitude of results is a speedometer graph, also known as a gauge graph. The scale of this graph is typically a semicircle that is

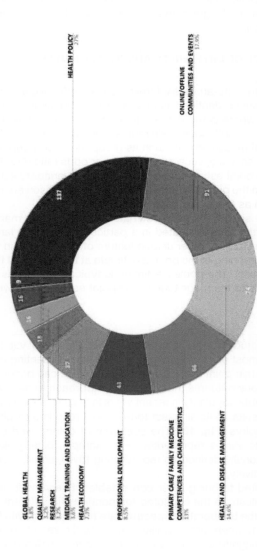

Fig. 7. Donut chart illustrating the proportion of health care–related hashtag themes in the realm of primary care and family medicine from a sample of 500 Twitter posts. The absolute frequency and the percentage of each theme are presented (note that 1.7%, n = 7, of the sample were not coded because they did not match any of the identified themes). (*From* Pinho-Costa L, Yakubu K, Hoedebecke K, et al. Healthcare hashtag index development: identifying global impact in social media. J Biomed Inform 2016;63:395; with permission.)

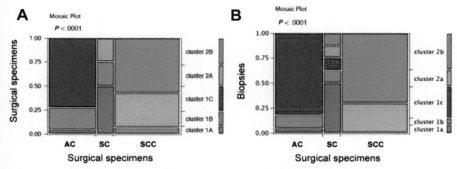

Fig. 8. Mosaic plots illustrating the proportion of different tumor subsets as identified via surgical specimens (*A*) and biopsies (*B*). AC, adenocarcinoma; SC, sarcomatoid carcinoma; SCC, squamous cell carcinoma. (*From* Pelosi G, Rossi G, Bianchi F, et al. Immunhistochemistry by means of widely agreed-upon markers (cytokeratins 5/6 and 7, p63, thyroid transcription factor-1, and vimentin) on small biopsies of non-small cell lung cancer effectively parallels the corresponding profiling and eventual diagnoses on surgical specimens. J Thorac Oncol 2011;6:1044; with permission.)

then labeled with appropriate values. A needle is often used to point to the value of the measure being graphed. A limitation of this approach is that only 1 value may be coherently graphed at a time.

A variation of the speedometer graph may be used to graph several correlation co-efficients simultaneously (**Fig. 12**). This may be useful when comparing an entire

Analysis 1. Exercise versus control

Study name	Sample size		Statistics for each study				Hedges's g and 95%CI	Relative weight
	Exercise	Control	Hedges's g	Lower limit	Upper limit	p-Value		
Blumenthal 1999	55	48	0,14	−0,25	0,52	·49		5,94
Blumenthal 2007	51	49	−0,29	−0,68	0,10	·15		5,91
Blumenthal 2012	15	9	−1,06	−1,91	−0,21	·01		3,72
Doyne 1987	13	11	−1,19	−2,04	−0,35	·01		3,75
Dunn 2005	17	13	−1,16	−1,92	−0,40	·00		4,11
Epstein 1986	7	10	−0,77	−1,72	0,18	·11		3,33
Foley 2008	8	5	−0,27	−1,32	0,77	·61		3,01
Gary 2010	18	15	−0,17	−0,84	0,50	·63		4,54
Hernat-Far 2012	10	10	−0,99	−1,89	−0,10	·03		3,55
Klein 1985	14	14	−0,22	−0,94	0,50	·55		4,29
Krogh 2009	47	42	−0,10	−0,51	0,31	·64		5,81
Krogh 2012	56	59	0,12	−0,24	0,49	·51		6,04
Martinsen 1985	24	19	−1,14	−1,77	−0,50	·00		4,69
Mota-Pereira 2011	19	10	−0,51	−1,26	0,25	·19		4,14
Mutrie 1986	9	7	−2,39	−3,64	−1,14	·00		2,42
Pilu 2007	10	20	−1,04	−1,82	−0,25	·01		4,01
Pinchasov 2000	9	9	−1,48	−2,49	−0,48	·00		3,15
Salehi 2014	20	20	−0,87	−1,51	−0,23	·01		4,70
Schuch 2011	15	11	−0,83	−1,62	−0,04	·04		4,00
Sims 2009	23	22	−0,53	−1,11	0,06	·08		4,95
Singh 1997	17	15	−1,75	−2,56	−0,95	·00		3,93
Singh 2005	18	19	−1,00	−1,67	−0,33	·00		4,53
Veale 1992	36	29	−0,33	−0,81	0,16	·19		5,45
	511	466	−0,68	−0,92	−0,44	·00		

−4,00   −2,00   0,00   2,00   4,00

Exercise   Control

Fig. 9. Forest plot of meta-analysis results evaluating the effects of exercise on the reduction of symptoms related to depression. The open squares represent the effect size point esti-mate for each of the included studies and the black diamond represents the pooled effect size across all included studies. (*From* Kvam S, Kleppe CL, Nordhus IH, et al. Exercise as a treatment for depression: a meta-analysis. J Affect Disord 2016;202:75; with permission.)

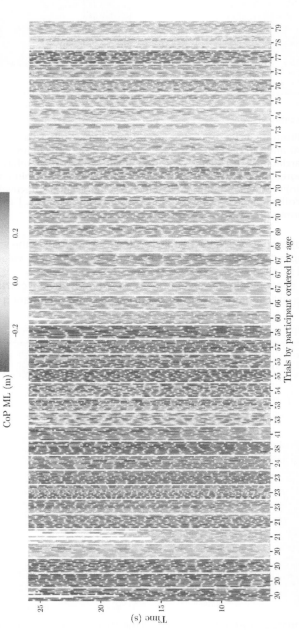

Fig. 10. Heat map of 400 stabilograms of mediolateral position of the center of pressure (CoP ML) during a balance test. The horizontal axis represents the trials per participant, with participants ordered by age. The vertical axis represents time during the trial, ranging from 6 to 26 seconds. The color scale for the position of CoP ML is at the top of the figure. (*From* Soancatl Aguilar V, van den Gronde J, Lamoth C, et al. Visual data exploration for balance quantification in real-time during exergaming. PLoS One 2017;12(1):e0170906; with permission.)

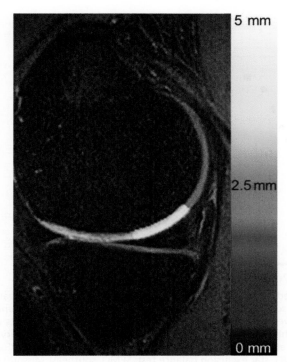

Fig. 11. Heat map depicting cartilage thickness on the medial femoral condyle. (*From* Schmitz RJ, Wang HM, Polprasert DR, et al. Evaluation of knee cartilage thickness: a comparison between ultrasound and magnetic resonance imaging methods. Knee 2017;24:219; with permission.)

matrix of dependent variables to each other. The midpoint of the gauge is labeled with a value of 0 (no correlation), whereas the far right end of the gauge is labeled with a value of +1.0 (perfect positive correlation), and the far left end is labeled with a value of −1.0 (perfect negative correlation). Symbols representing each pair of bivariate correlations are then placed on the graph to indicate the appropriate correlation coefficient point estimate. The basis for this type of figure is the Taylor diagram,[16] a more complex graph that is used to illustrate the correlation coefficient, root mean square error, and the SD between a modeled system and observed behavior. This described variation uses only the correlation coefficient portion of the Taylor diagram.

ILLUSTRATING TWO MEASURES SIMULTANEOUSLY
Dual Y-axis Graph

Investigators are often faced with the challenge of illustrating the results of more than 1 dependent measure within the context of a research study. Although each measure could be represented on a separate graph, this may cloud the relationships between the changes in multiple measures and is an inefficient use of space. One potential solution is the use of a graph with dual Y axes in which the Y axis on the left side of the graph is scaled for the primary outcome and the Y axis on the right side of the graph is scaled for the secondary outcome (**Fig. 13**). The X axis often consists of a time series. The 2 outcomes may be graphed in 1 of these combinations: (1) 1 as a bar graph and

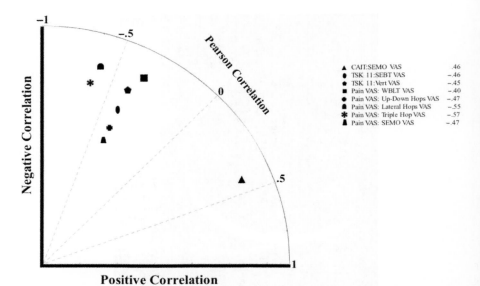

Positive Correlation

Fig. 12. A modified speedometer graph illustrating the magnitude of Pearson correlation coefficients from several correlation analyses comparing scores of self-reported questionnaires and perceived confidence scores when performing functional tests among a group of high school athletes with a history of ankle sprain. Note that the curved scale ranges from negative 1.0 at the top left to positive 1.0 at the bottom right. CAIT, Cumberland ankle instability tool; SEBT, star excursion balance test; SEMO, southeast Missouri agility test; TSK 11, Tampa scale of kinesiophobia 11; VAS, visual analog scale; Vert, vertical jump; WBLT, weight-bearing lunge test. Note: All reported *r* values are statistically significant; *P*<.05. This figure is derived from unpublished data (Revay O. Corbett, 2018) from the Exercise & Sport Injury Lab at the University of Virginia. (*Courtesy of* Revay O. Corbett, MS, ATC; with permission.)

the other as a line graph, (2) both as line graphs, and (3) both as bar graphs. Clear labeling of the axes and outcome measures is key to ensuring reader comprehension of these graphs.

Angle-Angle Plot

In musculoskeletal biomechanics research, it is common to simultaneously measure motion at more than 1 joint or in more than 1 plane at a single joint. An alternative to illustrating 2 streams of kinematic data independently is to plot them concurrently on an angle-angle plot (**Fig. 14**). One plane of motion is plotted on the X axis with the other plane on the Y axis. For each data sample, the kinematic values are plotted as in a scatterplot, and then a line is drawn to connect adjacent data points. Angle-angle plots are particularly effective for illustrating the coupling behavior of joint motions. A limitation of angle-angle plots is that there is not a time series on either axis, thus making it essential that the investigator clearly label important temporal events (eg, heel strike and toe-off during gait) on the graph.

Vector Graph

An effective manner of graphing simultaneous motion, or force, in 2 planes between 2 discrete time points is the use of vectors (**Fig. 15**). As in the angle-angle plot, 1

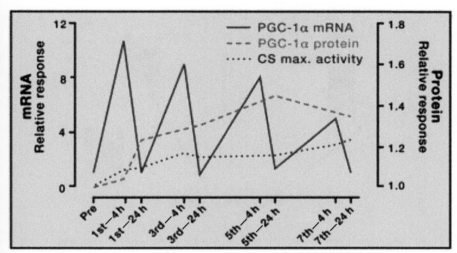

Fig. 13. A dual Y-axis graph with the scale for the relative response of mRNA (on the left Y axis) and protein (on the right Y axis) to 7 sessions of high-intensity interval training during a 2-week exercise intervention. Skeletal muscle biopsies from the vastus lateralis were obtained 4 hours and 24 hours after the first, third, fifth, and seventh training sessions. CS, citrate synthase; max, maximum; PGC-1α, peroxisome proliferator-activated receptor γ coactivator α. (*From* Hawley JA, Hargreaves M, Joyner MJ, et al. Integrative biology of exercise. Cell 2014;159(4):743; with permission.)

plane of motion is plotted on the X axis whereas a second plane of motion is plotted on the Y axis. Using a starting time point at the origin (0, 0 point) of the graph, the ending time point is plotted and the resultant vector is calculated. The length of the resultant vector represents the magnitude of coupled motion, whereas the angle of

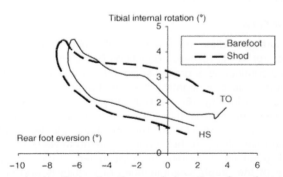

Fig. 14. An angle-angle plot illustrating the coupled motion of rearfoot inversion-eversion on the X axis and tibial internal-external rotation on the Y axis during the stance phase of running. Subjects ran in barefoot and shod conditions. Note that time is not depicted on either axis but the occurrence of heel strike (HS) and toe-off (TO) are clearly labeled on the graph to provide a temporal orientation. (*From* Eslami M, Begon M, Farahpour N, et al. Forefoot–rearfoot coupling patterns and tibial internal rotation during stance phase of barefoot versus shod running. Clin Biomech (Bristol, Avon) 2007;22:77; with permission.)

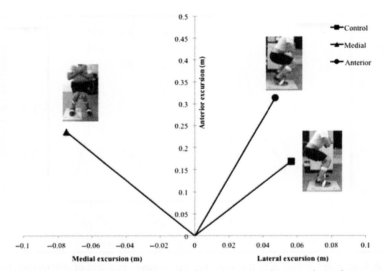

Fig. 15. This vector graph illustrates knee displacements simultaneously in the anterior and medial-lateral directions during squatting exercises performed with 3 different sets of instruction (control, anterior malaligned, and medial malaligned). The 0, 0 coordinate represents the starting position in upright stance whereas the position during maximal squat is represented by the symbols. (*From* Slater LV, Hart JM. The influence of knee alignment on lower extremity kinetics during squats. J Electromyogr Kinesiol 2016;31:98; with permission.)

the resultant vector from the horizontal indicates the ratio of motion between the 2 planes. The most common application of this type of analysis is called *vector coding* and is used to serially quantify the joint coupling behavior across movement tasks, such as gait.[17] It can, however, also be used to clearly graph coupled motion between any 2 discrete time points.

Receiver Operator Curve

In diagnostic accuracy studies, the estimation of sensitivity and specificity of diagnostic tests is central to the research questions being asked. For a diagnostic test that is scored on a continuous or ordinal scale, the establishment of threshold values for whether a test is positive or negative, the use of a receiver operator characteristic (ROC) curve can be helpful (**Fig. 16**). The ROC graph is constructed with sensitivity on the Y axis with values ranging from 0 to 1.0, whereas 1 minus specificity values on the X axis with values ranging from 0 to 1.0. This orientation places a test with both high sensitivity and high specificity in the upper left (or northwest) corner of the graph. There is also a diagonal line extending from the lower left hand corner to the upper right hand corner of the graph. Combinations of sensitivity and specificity that lie above that line are associated with diagnostic procedures with greater than a 50-50 chance of producing a correct diagnosis, whereas combinations below the line are less than chance.

To establish the best diagnostic threshold value, sensitivity and specificity are calculated at each possible threshold value in a data set. These combinations of values are then plotted on the ROC graph and a line is generated that extends from the lower left hand corner of the graph through each point plotted on the graph before

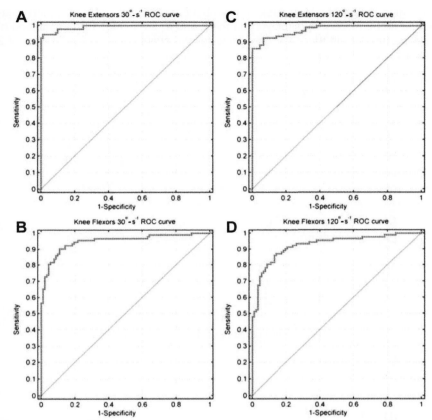

Fig. 16. A set of ROC curves of 4 decision rule models aimed at identifying feigned performance during maximal isokinetic strength testing. Note that the highest combination of sensitivity and specificity and the associated area under the curve values are found in descending order in graphs *A–D*. (*From* Almosnino S, Stevenson JM, Day AG, et al. Discriminating between maximal and feigned isokinetic knee musculature performance using waveform similarity measures. Clin Biomech (Bristol, Avon) 2012;27:381; with permission.)

culminating in the upper right hand corner of the graph. The point plotted in the most northwest position on the graph represents the optimal diagnostic threshold value and the area under the ROC curve represents the diagnostic accuracy of that threshold. The ROC curves of different diagnostic procedures may be compared on a single graph.

ILLUSTRATING THREE OR MORE MEASURES SIMULTANEOUSLY
Bubble Chart

A typical scatterplot graphs the scores of 2 measures, 1 on the X axis and the other on the Y axis, of individual subjects. The appearance of the symbols for each subject are typically uniform, although sometimes additional information can be conveyed, such as plotting the data of female subjects with filled circles and male subjects with clear circles. Bubble graphs expand on the simple scatterplot by changing the size of each subject's symbol based on the value of a third measure (the first 2 measures displayed on the X and Y axes) (**Fig. 17**). A limitation of simple scatterplots is that they only allow for the simultaneous presentation of 2 measures.

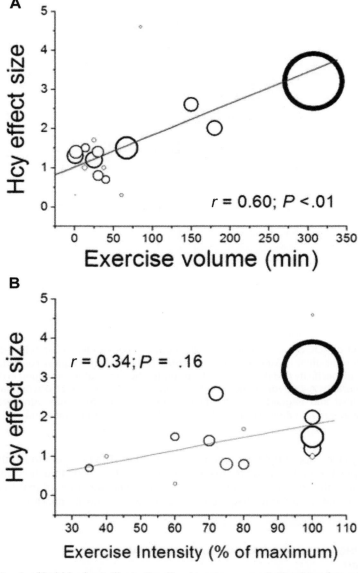

Fig. 17. A pair of bubble charts illustrating the dose-response relationship of exercise volume (*A*) and intensity (*B*) on the effect size changes of homocysteine (Hcy) across 18 separate studies. Each circle represents the results on a specific study and the size of the circle corresponds to the precision of each estimate to the fitted regression line. min, minutes. (*From* Deminice R, Ribeiro DF, Frajacomo FT. The effects of acute exercise and exercise training on plasma homocysteine: a meta-analysis. PLos One 2016;11(3):e0151653; with permission.)

3-D Scatterplot

Another useful way to visualize relationships between 3 different measures is the 3-D scatterplot (**Fig. 18**). The response variable is typically graphed on the Z axis whereas the 2 predictors variables are graphed on the X and Y axes. Software programs used to construct 3-D scatterplots typically allow for users to rotate the cube-shaped graph in an effort to find the best perspective for readers to see the direction and strength of the relationships between the 3 variables. Choosing a single 2-D view from which readers can view the graph on a static page in a printed article can be a challenge for investigators. Interactive graphing tools can counteract this challenge.

Radar Chart

A radar chart, also called a spider chart, may be used to simultaneously visualize the scores of 3 or more continuous or ordinal variables (**Fig. 19**). Each variable is plotted on its own spoke, or radius, extending outward from the center of the chart. The number of variables dictate the angle at which the spokes deviate from each other. Each spoke may have its own measurement scale although it can be confusing to readers when the scales differ. Measures from a single participant or group are plotted on each spoke and a line is then drawn to connect the scores of all measures. Results from additional participants and groups are then added to the chart, allowing for comparisons in the pattern of scores. Consideration should be given to the order in which the various outcome measures are displayed on the graph because differing orders can produce dissimilar shapes and lead to spurious interpretations of results.

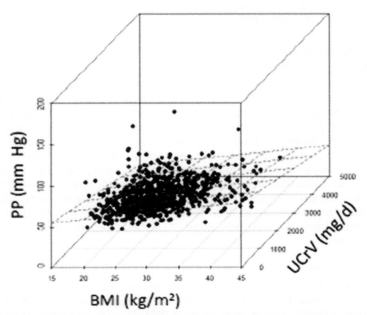

Fig. 18. A 3-D scatterplot illustrating the relationships between pulse pressure (PP), body mass index (BMI), and urinary creatinine excretion rate (UCrV) in 840 patients with chronic kidney disease. The red plane represents the plane of prediction for PP scores from BMI and UCrV scores. (*From* Shah PT, Martin R, Sanabria J, et al. Adiposity predicts pulse pressure in patients with chronic kidney disease: data from the modification of diet in renal disease. J Cardiol Curr Res 2016;7(2):00240; with permission.)

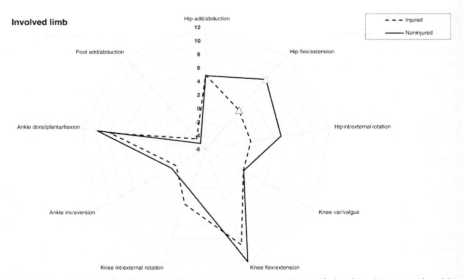

Fig. 19. A radar graph displaying the average joint position of the hip, knee, and ankle during a 20-second unipedal balance task for the involved limb in injured (ankle sprain) and uninjured groups. For each plane of motion, movements are listed in order of positive and negative values with neutral position equating to 0. Δ, statistically significant between-groups difference. (*From* Doherty C, Bleakley C, Hertel J, et al. Postural control strategies during single limb stance following acute lateral ankle sprain. Clin Biomech (Bristol, Avon) 2014;29:646; with permission.)

ILLUSTRATING DATA ACROSS TIME
Graphing Means and CIs Over Time

The visual presentation of time series data can present challenges, especially in regard to graphing variability estimates. One criticism of line graphs is that, similar to bar graphs, visualizing the distribution of individual participant scores within a data set can be difficult. When a time series consists of numerous measures taken at consistent intervals, 1 solution may be graphing 3 lines across the entire time series, with the middle line representative of the group mean and the top and bottom lines indicating the upper and lower boundaries of the associated CI around the mean. When this is done for 2 groups on the same graph, readers can visually assess the magnitude of differences in the group means as well as whether or not the CIs for the 2 groups overlap (**Fig. 20**). Some investigators specifically highlight the time epochs where the CIs do not overlap because these regions are often interpreted as significantly different from each other.

Time to Event Graph

Dichotomous outcomes, such as injury prevention (injured, not injured) or return to play after injury (returned, has not returned) are time series data typically assessed with survival analysis. Visualization of such data may be performed with Kaplan-Meier curves, where the follow-up time is expressed on the X axis and the proportion of participants who have or have not experienced the outcome of interest is displayed on the Y axis (**Fig. 21**). Group results showing the decline in the proportion of participants who not yet experienced the outcome of interest are plotted over time. The curves for 2 or more groups may be illustrated on the same graph for comparison.

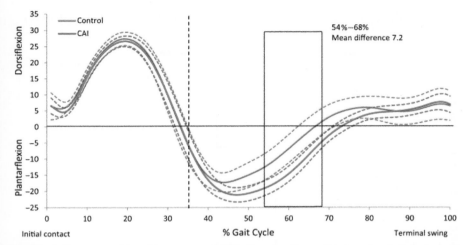

Fig. 20. A figure graphing the mean and 95% CI across the entire jogging gait cycle for a group with chronic ankle instability (CAI) and a healthy control group. The time points where the CIs for the 2 groups do not overlap are considered to be significantly different and are outlined in the rectangle. (*From* Chinn L, Dicharry J, Hertel J. Ankle kinematics of individuals with chronic ankle instability while walking and jogging on a treadmill in shoes. Phys Ther Sport 2013;14:236; with permission.)

Stacked Area Graph

An area graph is essentially a line graph with the area beneath the line filled in with color down to the X axis. The X axis is typically a time series. Area graphs may be a useful way to illustrate changes in a single measure over time. A limitation of area graphs is the lack of presentation of variability estimates.

If there is more than 1 category of data to be displayed on the same time series, a stacked area graph may be constructed to visualize the how the various categories change over time (**Fig. 22**). One limitation of stacked area graphs is that although the category shown on the bottom of the graph starts at the bottom of the measurement scale shown on the Y axis (usually 0); this first category's data are intuitive and easy to interpret. The other categories' scores, however, are stacked on top on another group's data and do not start at 0. Thus, stacked bar graphs may be better used for illustrating comparisons of proportional differences over time rather than comparison of absolute values in each category at each time point.

CAVEATS

The list of graph types described in this article are in no way meant to be all-inclusive. Other types of graphs may be more appropriate for illustrating a given set of results than those options discussed. In some cases, the best option may be a simple bar graph or line graph and investigators should be comfortable making that decision. This article is not a call for a permanent ban of all bar graphs and line graphs.

Readers must also be cognizant that the recommendations provided may become outdated with advances in data analytics and visualization. All the graphs described are static in nature and meant for the printed page. As more journals continue to move to online-only publications, investigators must recognize that journal articles at some point will move beyond the printed page (or PDF file) and possibilities like

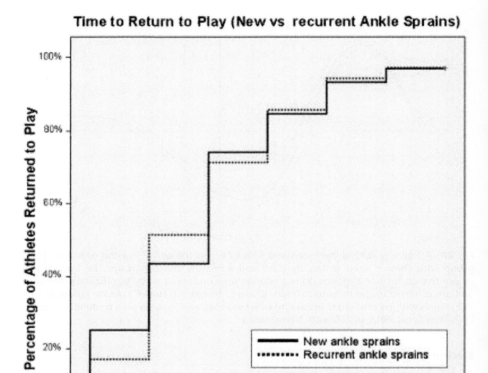

Fig. 21. A time to event graph illustrating the percentage of high school athletes who have returned to play at different time intervals after new versus recurrent ankle sprains. There was no significant difference in the return to play probabilities between these 2 groups. (*From* Medina McKeon JM, Bush HM, Reed A, et al. Return-to-play probabilities following new versus recurrent ankle sprains in high school athletes. J Sci Med Sport 2014;17:26; with permission.)

animated graphics and interactive figures may render many graphing techniques that are now accepted obsolete.[18]

RECOMMENDATIONS

The following recommendations are provided:

- A list of helpful graphing resources may be found in **Table 1**.
- Investigators should consider the importance of designing a signature figure for each research article they publish. Consider not only how this figure will look on the printed page but also how it will look on social media posts or on a slide presented by someone outside the research group.

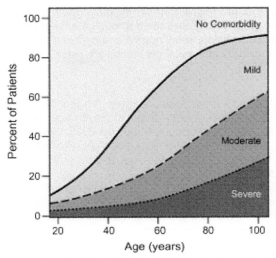

Fig. 22. A stacked area graph illustrating the percentage of 27,506 adult cancer patients with comorbidities across the age spectrum. (*From* Piccirillo JF, Vlahiotis A, Barrett LB, et al. The changing prevalence of comorbidity across the age spectrum. Crit Rev Oncol Hematol 2008;67:126; with permission.)

- Brainstorm multiple ways to graph a set of results before settling on how it will be done.
- Be cognizant of illustrating the results of individual participants and group distributions whenever possible.
- Clearly label each graph, paying particular attention to the labeling of the axes; the size, shape, and color of lines, bars, and other symbols; and how statistical significance and the magnitude of differences or strength of relationships are depicted.

Table 1
Selected resources to aid in making innovative graphs.

Resource	Website
Chart.js	www.chartjs.org
Creative Bloq	www.creativebloq.com/design-tools/data-visualization-712402
Data Hero	www.datahero.com
Matlab	www.mathworks.com
Microsoft Excel	www.support.office.com/en-us/excel
Plotly	www.plot.ly
R	www.r-project.org
RawGraphs	www.rawgraphs.io
SAS	www.sas.com
SPSS	www.spss.com
Tableau	www.tableau.com

Explore the following Web sites to learn more about using software packages and online tools for basic and advanced graphing functions. This list is not meant to be an all-inclusive list of graphing tools.

- Write a clear and informative caption for each graph in a manner that orients readers to the graph and guides them through the most important results.
- Prior to article submission, show graphs and captions to a colleague who is unfamiliar with the study and ask if the results are clearly presented.

REFERENCES

1. Anscombe FJ. Graphs in statistical analysis. Am Stat 1973;27:17–21.
2. Weissgerber TL, Milic NM, Winham SJ, et al. Beyond bar and line graphs: time for a new data presentation paradigm. PLoS Biol 2015;13(4):e1002128.
3. Schriger DL, Cooper RJ. Achieving graphical excellence: suggestions and methods for creating high-quality visual displays of experimental data. Ann Emerg Med 2001;37:75–87.
4. Cooper RJ, Schriger DL, Close RJ. Graphical literacy: the quality of graphs in a large-circulation journal. Ann Emerg Med 2002;40:317–22.
5. Lane DM, Sandor A. Designing better graphs by including distributional information and integrating words, numbers, and images. Psychol Methods 2009;14:239–57.
6. Paniello RC, Neely JG, Rich JT, et al. Practical guide to choosing an appropriate data display. Otolaryngol Head Neck Surg 2011;145:886–94.
7. Sperandei S. The pits and falls of graphical presentation. Biochem Med 2014;24:311–20.
8. Correll M, Gleicher M. Error bars considered harmful: exploring alternate encodings for mean and error. IEEE Trans Vis Comput Graph 2014;20:2142–51.
9. Duke SP, Bancken F, Crowe B, et al. Seeing is believing: good graphic design principles for medical research. Stat Med 2015;34:3040–59.
10. Rice K, Lumley T. Graphics and statistics for cardiology: comparing categorical and continuous variables. Heart 2016;102:349–55.
11. Weissgerber TL, Savic M, Winham SJ, et al. Data visualization, bar naked: a free tool for creating interactive graphics. J Biol Chem 2017;292:20592–8.
12. Nuzzo RL. The box plots alternative for visualizing quantitative data. PM R 2016;8:268–72.
13. Altman DG, Bland JM. Measurement in medicine: the analysis of method comparison studies. Statistician 1983;32:307–17.
14. Giavarina D. Understanding bland altman analysis. Biochem Med 2015;25:141–51.
15. Pelosi G, Rossi G, Bianchi F, et al. Immunhistochemistry by means of widely agreed-upon markers (cytokeratins 5/6 and 7, p63, thyroid transcription factor-1, and vimentin) on small biopsies of non-small cell lung cancer effectively parallels the corresponding profiling and eventual diagnoses on surgical specimens. J Thorac Oncol 2011;6:1039–49.
16. Taylor KE. Summarizing multiple aspects of model performance in a single diagram. J Geophys Res 2001;106:7183–92.
17. Herb CC, Chinn L, Dicharry J, et al. Shank-rearfoot joint coupling with chronic ankle instability. J Appl Biomech 2014;30:366–72.
18. Weissgerber TL, Garovic VD, Savic M, et al. From static to interactive: transforming data visualization to improve transparency. PLoS Biol 2016;14(6):e1002484.

Measuring Quality and Outcomes in Sports Medicine

Joseph J. Ruzbarsky, MD, Niv Marom, MD, Robert G. Marx, MD*

KEYWORDS

- Patient-reported outcome measures • Psychometric properties • Sports medicine
- Computer-adaptive testing

KEY POINTS

- Sports medicine contains an ever increasing array of available patient-reported outcome measures, which are commonly used metrics for assessing outcomes.
- Most traditional patient-reported outcome measures are constructed using classic test theory and are administered to patients as a whole, either on paper or digitally, for completion and score tabulation.
- Modern patient-reported outcomes measures, like the Patient-Reported Outcomes Measurement Information System, are constructed using item response theory and are amenable to computer-adaptive testing, which can decrease the question burden for patients and provide accurate results.

INTRODUCTION

Over the past several decades there has been a dramatic increase in the number of patient-reported outcome measures (PROMs) within medicine and orthopedics, specifically, as we have moved into an era of patient-centric care. PROMs have become so plentiful that it is difficult to keep track of the details of each instrument: how it is scored, for what conditions it was developed, and its intrinsic test characteristics or metrics.

A basic understanding of both the questionnaire content and the population for which it has been designed and tested is critical when collecting data for research purposes or for interpreting the published literature. When gathering data on patients,

Disclosure Statement: Dr R.G. Marx discloses his role as the Deputy Editor of Sports Medicine at the *Journal of Bone and Joint Surgery* and royalties from books published by Springer and Demos Health.
Conflicts of Interest and Source of Funding: There are no funding sources to disclose.
Department of Sports Medicine, Hospital for Special Surgery, 535 East 70th Street, New York, NY 10021, USA
* Corresponding author.
E-mail address: Marxr@hss.edu

choosing the single or few most appropriate instruments is important to accurately measure the outcomes of interest while minimizing the test burden for the patients. Furthermore, there may soon be a financial incentive to better understand PROMs, as they may potentially be linked to performance-based pay models after surgical procedures in the future.

With these important characteristics of PROMs in mind, the goals of this article are first to review some of the psychometric properties of these instruments and then to focus on the most commonly used PROMs within the realm of sports medicine, specifically focusing on the shoulder, elbow, knee, and hip joints. For the purposes of this review, measures focusing exclusively on lower extremity arthritis and general health measures, such as the 36-Item Short Form Health Survey (SF-36), are excluded.

BACKGROUND

Before a discussion about specific instruments, it is important to discuss the metrics used to quantify their intrinsic characteristics, also known as their psychometric properties. In general, the term *validity* is an index of how well a test measures what it is supposed to measure.[1,2] There are several types of validity that are used to describe an instrument. *Criterion or construct validity* is assessed by correlating the scores of the tool with that of a gold standard measure.[2] *Face validity* is when an expert in a specific field reviews the questions in the instrument and confirms that they measure the concept.[2] Finally, *content validity* measures whether the scale includes representative samples of the concept that the investigator is attempting to measure.[2]

Reliability is a measure of consistency or degree of dependability. In other words, reliability is the random error of a measure or the extent to which the scores are reproducible.[3] Reliability testing involves administration of an instrument at 2 time periods (usually days to weeks[2]) to the same individual and then determining the similarity of those responses. Agreement is then reported numerically in the form of the intraclass correlation coefficient (ICC). ICC values range from -1 to $+1$, with a value of 0 indicating only a random correlation. Internal consistency, reported by the Cronbach alpha, is another measure of reliability.[2] Cronbach alpha values range from 0 to 1, with values of 1 representing perfect internal consistency, which is a measure of the interitem correlation of all items in the scale. Values of 0.7 are generally considered acceptable.

Responsiveness is the ability of an instrument to detect clinical change over time. This value is measured by several statistics, including the responsiveness index (mean change score/variability of scores among subjects' scores); standardized response mean (mean change in score divided by the standard deviation of the change scores); or the effect size (mean change score divided by the standard deviation of baseline scores).

Minimal clinically important difference (MCID) is defined as the smallest difference in score in the domain of interest which patients perceive as beneficial.[4,5] Although values of MCIDs may not always be available or reported, a systematic review determined that under many circumstances, when patients with a chronic disease are asked to identify minimal change, the estimates fall very close to half a standard deviation of the results.[6]

Classic test theory is an instrument development theory whereby all of the questions of an instrument in combination is validated; this is in contrast to *item response theory* (IRT) whereby each item is independently validated.[7] Independent question validation allows for questions to be mixed and matched in administration and is required for computer adaptive testing.

Computer adaptive testing is a type of tailored testing whereby later questions depend on answers to earlier questions. This genre of testing is only possible in a computer or digitally based format.

The following paragraphs contains a summary of the most popular instruments used in sports medicine with each grouped by anatomic region. For the purposes of this review, the anatomic region is split up into hip (**Table 1**), knee (**Table 2**), shoulder (**Table 3**), elbow (**Table 4**), and miscellaneous.

HIP

The *Modified Harris Hip Score* (mHHS) consists of 8 questions (1 for pain and 7 for function) that are multiple choice and unequally weighted.[8] After final accumulation of scores a multiplier is used to scale the total score from 0 to 100. Higher scores indicate what is considered normal function.[8] This instrument is different from the Harris Hip Score (which is intended for use in a hip arthritis population) because the domains of deformity and range of motion were eliminated to create an instrument more applicable to a younger patient population who are candidates for hip arthroscopy rather than arthroplasty. This first description of the mHHS comes from a case series of patients who underwent hip arthroscopy whereby it was used as one of the outcome measures.[8]

The authors of the *Nonarthritic Hip Score* (NAHS) set out to create an instrument that focused on hip problems in a younger population.[9] This PROM was developed directly from the WOMAC (Western Ontario and McMaster Universities Osteoarthritis Index) score, which itself focuses on arthritic conditions of the hip and knee (50% of the questions in the NAHS come directly from the WOMAC). The 10 additional questions focus on either mechanical symptoms or activity level. The questionnaire contains 20 items, each equally weighted multiple choice with 1 to 5 answers providing a total score of 0 to 100, with 100 representing normal hip function.

The *Hip Outcome Score* (HOS) was specifically developed to fill a void among the available scales in the early 2000s with an intended patient population consisting of those with labral tears. It was designed to be useful throughout a wide range of activity levels because at the time of its inception, some of the other available PROMs were not built to differentiate participants in high-level activities and sports.[10] The scale was created through a collaboration between physicians and physical therapists, but notably there was no direct patient input in creating the scale.[11] The scale contains activities of daily living (ADLs) and sports subscales, each consisting of 5-point Likert scales with an option for *not applicable*. Answers of *not applicable* eliminate the question from scoring if there is a reason other than their hip problem that limits their activity, similar to the *Patellofemoral Pain Syndrome Severity Scale* (PFPS SS) scoring. The initial scale contained 28 total questions, but 2 were later removed after a preliminary trial in order to maintain unidimensionality.

The *International Hip Outcome Tool* (iHOT-33) was created by collaboration among the Multicenter Arthroscopy of the Hip Outcomes Research Network to focus on the evaluation of hip and groin disability in a young and physically active population.[11] The items were selected from existing instruments with additional items added on input from orthopedists, physical therapists, and patients. The cumulative item bank was then reduced using direct questions to orthopedic surgeons, who eliminated questions that were deemed unimportant or not useful. Each of its 33 questions is answered by means of a visual analog scale (VAS) and the total score is tabulated from 0 to 100, with higher scores representing a higher quality of life.

The *International Hip Outcome Tool 12*, analogous to the shortened version of the Disabilities of the Arm, Shoulder, and Hand (DASH), QuickDASH, is a shortened

Table 1
Patient-reported outcome measures of the hip

Instrument	Anatomic Region	Condition	Categories/Domains	Question Burden	Minimum Score	Maximum Score	Cronbach Alpha	ICC	MCID	Ref
Modified Harris Hip Score (mHHS)	Hip	Hip arthroscopy candidates	Pain and function	8	1	100	—	—	—	8
Nonarthritic Hip Score (NAHS)	Hip	Hip arthroscopy candidates	Function, mechanical symptoms, and activity	24	0	100	—	0.96	—	9
Hip Outcome Score (HOS)	Hip	—	ADLs and sports	26	0	200	0.96	—	6–9	10,51
International Hip Outcome Tool (iHOT-33)	Hip	Hip and groin disability	Symptoms, function, work, social/emotional/lifestyle	33	0	100	0.99	0.78	6	11
International Hip Outcome Tool-12 (iHOT-12)	Hip	—	Symptoms, function, work, social/emotional/lifestyle	12	0	100	—	0.89	—	12
Copenhagen Hip and Groin Outcome Score (HAGOS)	Hip	—	Symptoms, pain, ADLs, sports, quality of life	37	0	100	>0.78	—	—	13

Abbreviations: ADLs, activities of daily living; ref, reference.

Table 2
Patient-reported outcome measures of the knee

Instrument	Anatomic Region	Condition	Categories/Domains	Question Burden	Minimum Score	Maximum Score	Cronbach Alpha	ICC	MCID	Ref
AAOS Sports Knee Scale	Knee	—	Function, pain, activity limitation, and symptoms	23	0	100	0.86	0.92	—	3
Edinburgh Knee Function Scale	Knee	Nonsurgical knee problems	Pain and function	13	0	50	0.87	—	—	15
Functional Index Questionnaire (FIQ)	Knee	Patellofemoral knee pain	Function	8	0	16	0.48	0.85	—	16,17,52
Hospital for Special Surgery Pediatric Functional Activity Brief Scale (HSS Pedi-FABS)	Knee	—	Activity level	8	0	30	0.91	0.91	—	30
International Knee Documentation Committee (IKDC) Subjective Knee Form	Knee	—	Symptoms, sports and activities, and function	18	0	100	0.77–0.97	0.87–0.99	6.3–16.7	18,19,51

(continued on next page)

Table 2
(continued)

Instrument	Anatomic Region	Condition	Categories/Domains	Question Burden	Minimum Score	Maximum Score	Cronbach Alpha	ICC	MCID	Ref
Knee Injury and Osteoarthritis Outcome Score (KOOS)	Knee	ACL and meniscal injuries	Pain, symptoms, and function	42	0	100	—	0.75–0.93	8–10	20,51
Knee Outcomes Survey - Activities of Daily Living (KOS-ADL)	Knee	—	Symptoms and function	17	0	100	0.89–0.98	0.94–0.98	—	19,21
Knee Quality of Life 26-Item (KQL-26)	Knee	Ligamentous or meniscal injury	Function	26	0	100	0.91	—	—	22
Knee Self-Efficiency Scale (K-SES)	Knee	ACL injuries	Activities and function tasks	22	0	220	0.94	0.75	—	23
Kujala Anterior Knee Pain Scale (KAKPS)	Knee	Patellofemoral knee pain	Symptoms	13	0	100	—	—	—	25,52,53
Lysholm Knee Score	Knee	ACL tears	Symptoms and function	8	0	100	0.65–0.73	0.87–0.97	—	19,26
Marx Activity Rating Scale	Knee	—	Activity level	4	0	16	—	0.97	—	27
Patellofemoral Pain Syndrome Severity Scale (PFPS SS)	Knee	Patellofemoral knee pain	Pain and function	10	0	100	—	—	—	31

Abbreviation: ACL, anterior cruciate ligament.

Table 3
Patient-reported outcome measures of the shoulder

Instrument	Anatomic Region	Condition	Categories/Domains	Question Burden	Minimum Score	Maximum Score	Cronbach Alpha	ICC	MCID	Ref
Shoulder pain and disability index (SPADI)	Shoulder	—	Pain and disability	13	0	100	0.95	0.65	—	34
American Shoulder and Elbow Surgeons Evaluation Form (ASES)	Shoulder and elbow	—	Pain and function	11	0	100	—	—	6.6 (all conditions); 12–17 (rotator cuff disease)	36,54,55
Disabilities of the Arm, Shoulder, and Hand (DASH)	Upper extremity	—	Symptoms and functional status	30	0	100	—	0.77–0.98	10 (shoulder)	38,39
QuickDASH	Upper extremity	—	Symptoms and functional status	11	0	100	>0.92	>0.94	—	5,39
The Shoulder Rating Questionnaire (SRQ)	Shoulder	—	Pain, activities, satisfaction, and improvement	20	17	100	0.86	—	12	1
The Simple Shoulder Test (SST)	Shoulder	—	Function	12	0	12	—	0.97–0.99	2.4	37,40,54
Western Ontario Shoulder Instability Index (WOSI)	Shoulder	Shoulder instability	Physical symptoms, sports and recreation, work, lifestyle, emotions	21	0	100	—	0.91–0.95	10.4	41,54,55

(continued on next page)

Table 3
(continued)

Instrument	Anatomic Region	Condition	Categories/Domains	Question Burden	Minimum Score	Maximum Score	Cronbach Alpha	ICC	MCID	Ref
The Western Ontario Osteoarthritis of the Shoulder Index (WOOSI)	Shoulder	Shoulder OA	Pain and physical symptoms; sport, recreation, and work; lifestyle function; and emotional function	19	0	100	—	0.96	—	42
Western Ontario Rotator Cuff Index (WORC)	Shoulder	Rotator cuff tears	Physical symptoms, sports and recreation, work, lifestyle, and emotions	21	0	100	—	0.96	11.7	35,54,55
The Rotator Cuff Quality of Life Measure (RC-QOL)	Shoulder	Rotator cuff tears	Symptoms/physical complaints, sports/recreation; work-related concerns; lifestyle; and social/emotional	34	0	100	—	—	—	43
Oxford Shoulder Scores (OSS)	Shoulder	—	Pain, function, emotional	12	12	60	—	0.89–0.92	—	45
Single Assessment Numeric Evaluation (SANE)	Shoulder	—	NA	1	0	100	—	—	—	46
Shoulder Activity Level (SAL)	Shoulder	—	Activity level	7	9	20	—	0.92	—	47

Abbreviations: NA, not applicable; OA, osteoarthritis; ref, reference.

Table 4
Patient-reported outcome measures of the elbow

Instrument	Anatomic Region	Condition	Categories/Domains	Question Burden	Minimum Score	Maximum Score	Cronbach Alpha	ICC	MCID	Ref
Oxford elbow score (OES)	Elbow	—	Pain, symptoms, and activity	12	0	100	—	—	—	48
Patient-rated Elbow Evaluation (PREE)	Elbow	—	Pain and function	22	0	100	—	0.95	—	49,56
American Shoulder and Elbow Surgeons Evaluation Form-e (ASES-e)	Shoulder and elbow	—	Pain, function, and satisfaction	11	0	100	—	0.64–0.95	—	36,56
Disabilities of the Arm, Shoulder, and Hand (DASH)	Upper extremity	—	Symptoms and functional status	30	0	100	0.97	0.92–0.97	17 (elbow)	38,39,56
QuickDASH	Upper extremity	—	Symptoms and functional status	11	0	100	>0.92	>0.94	—	5,39,56

Abbreviation: ref, reference.

version containing only about 30% of the iHOT-33.[12] The goal for this abridged version is to reduce questionnaire fatigue and to allow for ease of use in both the initial assessment and the follow-up in clinical practice as opposed to the iHOT-33, which was developed for use in clinical research.[11] The 12 items were chosen based on a sample of more than 1800 patients who had completed the iHOT-33. The investigators found that only 4 items accounted for 99% of the variability in iHOT-33 scores. Combining these items with regression analysis results, domain memberships, and frequency-importance products led to the creation of a 12-item questionnaire. Similar to the iHOT-33, each question is equally weighted and answered by means of a VAS. The investigators found that this 12-item version captured about 95% of the variability seen in the iHOT-33.

The *Copenhagen Hip and Groin Outcome Score* was introduced in 2011 and developed for young to middle-aged, physically active individuals with long-standing hip and/or groin pain but lacking any specific diagnosis.[13] It was developed completely using the Consensus-Based Standards for the Selection of Health Status Measurement Instruments checklist.[14] For item generation, the investigators relied on a systematic review of the literature, a focus group of experts, and patient interviews. They decided to use the HOOS (Hip disability and Osteoarthritis Outcome Score) as a template for development of their instrument because of its ease of use, self-explanatory nature, and widespread adoption. They also added 3 items from the HOS. Because the two contributing instruments focused exclusively on the hip, the investigators modified each item to also include the groin by replacing the word *hip* with the phrase *hip and/or groin* in each item. A prospective clinical trial involving 50 patients was used to determine the specifications of the instrument in addition to narrowing the total questions to 37. Each question is graded from 0 (none) to 4 (extreme), and the total score is calculated to fall among 0 to 100. Analysis revealed that the instrument did not have any significant ceiling and floor effects except in the physical activity and ADL subscales.

KNEE

The *AAOS Sports Knee Scale,* introduced by the American Academy of Orthopedic Surgeons (AAOS) in 1998, builds on 5 separate lower limb instruments. Development of this instrument began in 1994 at a joint meeting between the AAOS and the Council of Musculoskeletal Specialty Societies.[3] The sports-knee questionnaire was initially piloted on a cohort of 59 patients with a variety of knee injuries. It contains 23 questions focusing on symptoms, activity, and pain. It is scored on a 100-point scale.[3]

The *Edinburgh Knee Function Scale* was first reported in 1999 with the intended population of patients with knee complaints not requiring surgical intervention.[15] The investigators acquired items primarily from 2 sources: the Lysholm rating scale and the Aberdeen Low Back Pain scale. In total it contains 13 questions each with 4 to 6 multiple choice responses. Total scores range from 0 to 50 with higher scores indicating a more severely affected state.[15]

The *Functional Index Questionnaire* was developed in the 1980s and was designed to assess patellofemoral syndrome.[16] The scale contains 8 questions all relating to function. Each question can be answered with the following responses: *unable to do, can do with problem*, and *no problem*. Unfortunately, the reliability of this test was found to be poor with an ICC of 0.483, thought to be a consequence of the often paroxysmal nature of PF pain.[17]

The *International Knee Documentation Committee Subjective Knee Form* (IKDC) was developed "to detect improvement or deterioration in symptoms, function, and sports activity experienced by patients with a variety of knee conditions."[18] This questionnaire underwent several iterations after incorporating the results of testing patient groups. Its final version included a total of 18 questions. The questions are all equally weighted, as these were found to correlate very highly with other weighting methods with added simplicity. Total scores are normalized from 0 to 100, with higher scores indicating lower symptoms and higher function. In its entirety, the instrument takes patients approximately 10 minutes to complete and contains simple language; several translations exist to expand its use.[19] Its minimal detectable change was determined to be between 8 and 16 points.[19]

The *Knee Injury and Osteoarthritis Outcome Score* was constructed from literature review, expert panel, and pilot study.[20] It is intended for patients with anterior cruciate ligament (ACL) and meniscal injuries and their related treatment.[20] This instrument contains the WOMAC questionnaire in its entirety because the investigators decided that measuring and detecting arthritis, a potential long-term complication of this injury, was determined to be an important outcome to capture in this patient population. Each question is answered by means of 5-item Likert scales. Scoring is equally weighted with total scores converted to a 100-point scale. A score of 0 represents those that are most severely affected. It takes patients approximately 10 minutes to complete.[19]

The *Knee Outcome Survey-Activities of Daily Living* instrument, proposed by Irrgang and colleagues[21] in 1998, was designed to address the functional limitations in both performing ADLs and athletic activities. Its items were chosen from several preexisting scales with the goal of representing issues reported by patients with a variety of knee pathologies: ligamentous or meniscal injuries, patellofemoral pain, or osteoarthritis. The score itself consists of 17 multiple choice questions, each equally weighted and scored from 0 to 100. Its respondent burden is approximately 5 minutes.[19]

The *Knee Quality of Life 26-item Questionnaire* was created to provide an instrument specific for ligamentous or meniscal injury of the knee focusing on knee-related quality of life, as its name suggests.[22] Its items were generated exclusively from the patients' perspective relying on patient interviews, focus groups, and follow-up interviews. It consists of 26 items, each scored numerically from 0 to 4. Each question is equally weighted to generate total scores from 0 to 100, with 100 representing the best possible quality of life. In its initial testing, it correlated most highly with the Lysholm score.[22]

The *Knee Self-Efficiency Scale* is quite different than many of the other questionnaires because instead of measuring qualities, such as symptoms and function, it was developed in 2005 to evaluate patient-perceived self-efficacy.[23] Self-efficacy is thought to influence how well one ultimately copes with and eventually overcomes recovery from a major obstacle, in this case after ACL injuries.[24] The items were developed by a group of physical therapists, orthopedic surgeons, and medical physicians. After 2 separate pilot studies, it was reduced to 22 items. Each item is scored on a 0 to 10 Likert scale with 0 representing *not at all certain* and 10 representing *very certain*. Total scores range from 0 to 220, with higher scores representing complete certainty.

The *Kujala Anterior Knee Pain Scale* was the first instrument developed specifically for disorders of the patellofemoral compartment.[25] The investigators set out in 1993 to define the questions that are most important for representing all types of patellofemoral disorders, including overuse, traumatic, acute, or chronic. The instrument consists of 13 multiple choice questions each unequally weighted, which generates a cumulative score of 0 to 100. As part of the investigators' initial description of the scale, they performed a knee MRI, which examined the patellofemoral compartment, and aimed to correlate some of the questions with MRI findings. They found that the overall score correlated best with the measured lateral patellar tilt seen with the quadriceps extended and the knee flexed.[25]

The *Lysholm Knee Scale* was designed for "knee ligament injuries."[26] The investigators point out that some of the novelty of this scale was due to the addition of questions grading instability symptoms. They assess instability with items containing the term *giving way* that differentiated it from some of the other scales available at that time. The questionnaire contains 8 unequally weighted multiple choice questions, which result in a total score ranging from 0 to 100. Higher scores indicate less pathologic states.

Unlike most of the other PROMs present in this review, the initial purpose of the *Marx Activity Rating Scale* was not to measure the outcomes after medical or surgical interventions.[27] The investigators specifically set out to quantify activity levels. Activity levels can be prognostic of future expectations after an injury but are also critical to quantify whenever performing comparisons between groups.[27] It was developed because the investigator thought the only existing activity scale (the Tegner) was completely sport specific, which was associated with some limitations.[27] Initial item generation was accomplished through interviews with orthopedists, athletic trainers, physical therapists, and patients. The final instrument resulted from surveying patients with a variety of knee problems about both the importance and physical difficulty in performing specific maneuvers. Only those actions determined to be both the most important and the most difficult to perform were included. It resulted in a 4-question scale that could be completed in less than 1 minute. Total scores range from 0 to 16, with 16 representing the highest activity levels.

The *Tegner Activity Scale* is another activity grading scale that was created in 1985 as a complement to functional scales for knee ligamentous injuries.[28] The investigators point out that an activity scale is necessary because "limitations in knee function may be masked by an involuntarily low activity level."[28] The scale itself is a Gutmanmethod scale, unlike most of the other PROMs in this review, which are multi-item responses.[28] Gutman-style scales consist of a hierarchical arrangement in which any single item subsumes and differs in score than those below it.[29] It is made up of 10 levels. Level 10 represents the highest and consists of the "soccer - national and international elite" and 0, the lowest, representing "sick leave or disability pension because of knee problems."[28] This scale takes patients approximately 3 minutes to complete.[19]

The *Hospital for Special Surgery Pediatric Functional Activity Brief Scale* was developed in 2013 to fill the void of objective assessment of activity levels in adolescents from 10 to 18 years old, as the existing scales at the time were designed for adults.[30] The investigators performed a systematic review at the time of publication and found only 2 pediatric PROMs focusing on activity level.[30] Items were generated through the expert opinions of 2 pediatric and 1 sports medicine orthopedic surgeons in addition to responses from 20 patients who were surveyed. A separate group of 20 patients were then used for item reduction, another 20 for pilot testing, and finally 51 for validation of the instrument. In total the instrument contains 8 multiple choice questions, each scoring between 0 and 3 or 0 and 4, with total scores ranging from 0 to 30, with higher scores indicating higher activity levels. In 6 of the 8 questions it specifically asks about activity levels over the last month. The instrument's questions are written at a 6.6-year reading level; but for validation, parents were allowed to assist children younger than 13 years. The ceiling and floor effects are 3.9% and 0%, respectively.[30]

Item generation for the PFPS SS began with a literature review and then was modified after input from both clinicians and patients.[31] One of the creator's goals was to develop a scale focusing on patellofemoral complaints for use in an athletic or military population.[31] It is made up of 2 subscales focusing on pain and function and was modified after pilot testing to result in 10 total questions, each of which are answered by means of a VAS. Questions are answered based on the greatest amount of pain experienced over the past week. The goal of asking questions in this manner is to improve the evaluation of symptoms related to this condition, which often wax and wane. Scoring of this instrument is unique. Questions can be eliminated if patients do not partake in the specified activities, and in those cases the maximum score will be based on an adjusted denominator. A maximum score, however, will be assigned for that question if that specific item is avoided because of pain. The total score is then normalized to 100%.

The *Quality of Life Outcome Measure for Chronic ACL Deficiency* was developed in the late 1990s and focuses on measuring quality of life in patients with chronic ACL deficiency. Item generation was achieved through a literature review in addition to expert opinions from primary care sports medicine physicians, orthopedic surgeons, trainers, and physical therapists.[32] Items are divided into 5 separate domains. After pilot testing, the total number of questions was reduced to 32. Each question is answered by means of a VAS. Total scores can range from 0 to 100. In the original report of this instrument, the construct validity was determined from testing this questionnaire on 50 consecutive patients with chronic ACL deficiency. The mean score of those indicated for surgery was 31, whereas those pursuing nonoperative treatments was 79.

The *Western Ontario Meniscal Evaluation Tool* was developed with the goal of creating a disease-specific health-related quality-of-life outcome measure focusing on meniscal pathologic conditions.[33] The instrument was developed and refined using a cohort of patients with symptoms of swelling, catching, or locking with MRI evidence of meniscal pathology. Item generation was accomplished through direct patient input. Items were later modified to an eighth-grade reading level. The instrument contains 16 equally weighted items scored by means of a VAS, with total scores ranging from 0 to 100. The floor effect was determined to be 5.7% and the ceiling 1.7%.

SHOULDER

The *Shoulder Pain and Disability Index* was developed in 1991.[34] After item reduction based on poor test-retest reliability or a low correlation with shoulder range of motion on the involved side in a cohort of 37 male outpatients with various causes of shoulder pain,[35] the final instrument was trimmed to 13 total items. Each item is answered by means of a 0 to 10 VAS. The cumulative score is then converted to a 0 to 100 scale with 0 corresponding to the best possible score. The instrument contains 2 major categories: pain and disability.

The *American Shoulder and Elbow Surgeons Evaluation Form* (ASES) was developed over a 3-year period from 1990 to 1993 with the initial goals of ease of use, a method of assessing ADLs, and inclusion of a patient self-evaluation section.[36] The scale consists of a patient-reported and physician-evaluated sections built to evaluate pain, instability, and ADLs. The authors focus only on the PRO section, as that portion of the instrument can be applied independently. In this section, the pain and ADL portions are equally weighted in generating the final score. The pain portion consists of only a single VAS pain scale and is worth 50% of the total score. The 10 function-based questions have 4 possible responses from 0 (*unable to*) to 3 (*not difficult*) and are averaged to consist of the other 50% of the total score.[36] The MCID was determined in a later study to be 20.9.[37]

The DASH questionnaire was developed in 1996 to be used as both a research and clinical practice tool to evaluate symptoms and functional status of any upper extremity musculoskeletal condition.[38] The goal of this measure was to be able to develop an outcome measure that would have broad applicability and, thus, allow for comparisons across several upper extremity conditions.[38] The investigators pooled items from 13 different existing upper extremity instruments to generate the final questionnaire.[39] In total, the instrument is made up of 30 items, 23 of which focus on function; the final 7 focus on pain and other symptoms. Each question has 5 options and is graded on a 0 to 100 scale, with higher scores indicating more severe symptoms and functional deficits.

The *QuickDASH* was introduced nearly a decade after the DASH as a shortened form of the 30 question questionnaire.[39] The authors calculated that reducing the DASH to 11 items using a formula for the Spearman-Brown prophesy would still ensure a Cronbach alpha value for the shortened instrument of 0.90 to 0.95.[39] Three separate item reduction techniques were then used to reduce the number of items to 11. The concept-retention technique, in which items from each domain were subjectively chosen to be retained in order to maintain the theoretic framework of the original instrument, was chosen. In the end items focusing on weakness, stiffness, family care, sexual activities, and self-image were eliminated. Formal metric analysis found that this version resulted in an instrument most similar to the DASH ($r = 0.98$), and therefore, this version was chosen as the QuickDASH. Like the DASH it is scored from 0 to 100 with higher scores representing greater disability.

The *Shoulder Rating Questionnaire* was reported in 1997 and developed on a group of patients with a variety of disorders of the shoulder. It consists of several of domains: pain, activities of daily living, recreational activities, work, satisfaction, and a global assessment.[1] The global assessment domain consists of just a single VAS but the remaining domains are made up of multiple choice questions with answers ranging from *poorest* to *best*. For calculating the total score, each domain is weighted differently based on "consultation with several shoulder surgeons and patients regarding the relative importance of each of the domains."[1] The pain domain is weighted the heaviest (maximum score: 40 points), and the work domain is weighted the lowest (maximum score: 10 points). The total score can range from 17 to 100 points. The investigators that introduced the scale hypothesized that an improvement of 12 points between preoperative and postoperative scores was clinically important.[1]

The *Simple Shoulder Test* (SST) is an instrument designed at the University of Washington that builds upon items contained in the ASES in order to create a 12-item functional assessment tool.[40] Each item is a yes or no question. In the initial article that describes the development of this instrument, the investigators explain how it was tested both in a cohort of patients with normal shoulders and then in a variety of cohorts of patients with different pathologic states. They demonstrated near-ceiling effects in the normal cohort and then various degrees of decreased performance in their pathologic cohorts. The MCID was determined to be 2.4.[37]

The *Western Ontario Shoulder Instability Index* (WOSI) is one of the several disease-specific instruments developed at the University of Western Ontario. It is made up of 5 domains: physical symptoms, sports and recreation, work, lifestyle, and emotions.[41] Items for the scale were initially chosen through interviews with 33 patients and their spouses about ways instability affected the patients' quality of life. This process resulted in a total of 291 initial items, which were then subsequently reduced to 21 items, each equally weighted and answered by means of a VAS. The instrument is designed for an eighth-grade reading level. The total score can vary from 0 (best) to 2100 (worst). It comes with an appendix that participants can refer to should questions arise when completing the questionnaire. In the initial description and testing of the scale, it was determined to be more responsive than both the DASH and the ASES.[41]

The *Western Ontario Osteoarthritis of the Shoulder Index* was developed using the same process as the WOSI by the same investigators and out of the same institution in 2001.[42] The population targeted included those with symptomatic osteoarthritis of the shoulder. It contains 19 questions from a variety of domains: pain and physical symptoms; sport, recreation, and work; lifestyle function; emotional function.[42]

The *Western Ontario Rotator Cuff Index* (WORC) is both a disease- and joint-specific instrument from the Western Ontario group focusing on rotator cuff pathology and was introduced in 2003.[35] The instrument was initially assessed in patients who were being treated for rotator cuff tendinosis with no or small full-thickness cuff tears. It contains 5 domains: physical symptoms, sports and recreation, work, lifestyle, and emotions. The WORC correlated most strongly with the ASES ($r = 0.68$) and the DASH ($r = 0.63$).[35]

The *Rotator Cuff Quality of Life Measure* (RC-QOL)[43] like the WORC is also rotator cuff specific. Item generation was determined in a manner similar to the WORC, ultimately resulting in 34 items each answered by means of a VAS.[44] It contains 5 domains, including symptoms and physical complaints, sports and recreation, work-related concerns, lifestyle issues, and social and emotional issues. In the index study reporting this PROM, the investigators reported a follow-up study in which 86 patients with either large or massive randomized controlled trials with greater than a 2-year follow-up who underwent surgery and had the RC-QOL, ASES, and SF-36 administered. They found that the RC-QOL scores were significantly higher in the large cohort as compared with the massive tears, and the score was best correlated with the ASES.[43]

The *Oxford Shoulder Scores* was developed out of Oxford University in the early 1990s with the goal of assessing the outcomes of operations on the shoulder but excluding stabilization procedures.[45] The questionnaire contains 12 equally weighted items each scored from 1 to 5 producing total scores of 12 (least difficulties) to 60 (most difficulties).[45] The investigators reported good internal consistency (ICC 0.98–0.92) and reproducibility and correlated best with the Stanford Health Assessment questionnaire and the Constant score.[45]

Single Assessment Numeric Evaluation is a single-question instrument: How would you rate your shoulder today as a percentage of normal? It was proposed in 1999, and the response is a 0% to 100% scale. In the index article, the investigators compared it with the Rowe (mixed clinician and patient-reported questionnaire) and the combined patient and clinician ASES scores.[46] The investigators found that it was the most time-efficient PROM and that it correlated well with the two other scores ($r = 0.77$ with Rowe and $r = 0.69$ with ASES) in patients presenting with a diverse range of shoulder instability operations.[46]

Finally, in contrast to many of the other aforementioned shoulder-specific PROMs, the *Shoulder Activity Level* score was developed in order to focus on upper extremity activity levels as opposed to symptoms and function.[47] Items were generated by interviewing patients with a variety of shoulder pathologies at various points in treatment and practitioners. The score contains 5 items, each scored on a 5-point scale from 0 (*never performed*) to 4 (*performed daily*) for a total score of 0 to 20. The patients are asked to choose an answer "that reflects a frequency consistent with their healthiest, most active state during the last year."[47] In addition to the numeric score, patients can also receive a 2-letter score based on their responses to 2 multiple choice questions: Do you participate in contact sports? Do you participate in sports that involve hard overhand throwing, overhand serving, or lap/distance swimming?: (A) no; (B) yes, without organized officiating; (C) yes, with organized officiating; or (D) yes, at a professional level (ie, paid to play). The instrument had good correlation with the SST (r = 0.46) and the Marx Activity Scale (r = 0.66).[47]

ELBOW

The *Oxford Elbow Score* was developed for patients undergoing any operation on their elbow.[48] It consists of 12 items, each multiple choice with 5 options. It is broken down into 3 domains: pain, functional impairment, and participation in activities and psychological aspects of condition. Scores range from 0 to 100. In initial testing, it was found to positively correlate with the Mayo elbow score, the DASH, and the SF-36.

The *Patient-Rated Elbow Evaluation* was adopted from the *Patient-Rated Wrist Evaluation*.[49] It was developed "using a variety of elbow complaints"[49] in 70 patients. It consists of a 20-item pain subscale and 2 function subscales (specific activities and role performance). Each item is scored from 0 to 10 resulting in cumulative scores of 0 to 100, with higher scores corresponding to greater pain and disability.

PATIENT-REPORTED OUTCOMES MEASUREMENT INFORMATION SYSTEM

The *Patient-Reported Outcomes Measurement Information System* (PROMIS) was developed as part of a National Institutes of Health Roadmap program with the goal of developing an efficient state-of-the-art assessment system for self-reported health. It is an IRT as opposed to an instrument based on classical test theory in that each question is independently validated.[7] The test itself is plastic; it offers the ability to generate an array of possible combinations of items based on a respondent's previous responses to questions. The advantage of this type of instrument is that the amount of questions required to generate a score can be significantly reduced, the instrument can have greater accuracy, results can be reported in terms of a T-score, which is universally and consistently understandable and can result in a broad score range with limited ceiling and floor effects.[7] Within orthopedics alone, the PROMIS has already been evaluated and validated within the subspecialties of foot and ankle, upper extremity, trauma, sports medicine, and spine. Within sports medicine, the PROMIS physical function computer adaptive testing (CAT) instrument was found to correlate highly with the IKDC for postoperative ACL reconstruction while demonstrating greater responsiveness.[7,50]

SUMMARY

A thorough understanding is required for those intending to use and interpret PROMs for research or clinical care. Most older questionnaires are disease specific or anatomically focused and were developed according to classic test theory. New instruments, such as the PROMIS, are constructed using item response theory. Constructed in this manner, these new measures have the potential for computer-adaptive testing, which has the potential to change the way these tests are adopted and administered.

REFERENCES

1. L'Insalata JC, Warren RF, Cohen SB, et al. A self-administered questionnaire for assessment of symptoms and function of the shoulder. J Bone Joint Surg Am 1997;79(5):738–48. Available at: http://www.ncbi.nlm.nih.gov/entrez/query.fcgi?cmd=Retrieve&db=PubMed&dopt=Citation&list_uids=9160947.
2. Marx RG. Knee rating scales. Arthroscopy 2003;19(10):1103–8.

3. Johanson NA, Liang MH, Daltroy L, et al. American Academy of Orthopaedic Surgeons lower limb outcomes assessment instruments: reliability, validity, and sensitivity to change. J Bone Joint Surg Am 2004;86A(5):902–9. Available at: http://search.ebscohost.com/login.aspx?direct=true&db=cin20&AN=2005026784&site=ehost-live.

4. Jaeschke R, Singer J, Guyatt GH, et al. Measurement of health status ascertaining the minimal clinically important difference. Control Clin Trials 1989;10:407–15.

5. Franchignoni F, Vercelli S, Giordano A, et al. Minimal clinically important difference of the disabilities of the arm, shoulder and hand outcome measure (DASH) and its shortened version (QuickDASH). J Orthop Sports Phys Ther 2014;44(1):30–9.

6. Norman GR, Sloan JA, Wyrwich KW. Interpretation of changes in health-related quality of life: the remarkable universality of half a standard deviation. Med Care 2003;41(5):582–92.

7. Brodke DJ, Saltzman CL, Brodke DS. PROMIS for orthopaedic outcomes measurement. J Am Acad Orthop Surg 2016;24(11):744–9.

8. Byrd JWT, Jones KS. Prospective analysis of hip arthroscopy with 2-year follow-up. Arthroscopy 2000;16(6):578–87.

9. Christensen CP, Althausen PL, Mittleman MA, et al. The nonarthritic hip score: reliable and validated. Clin Orthop Relat Res 2003;406:75–83.

10. Martin RL, Kelly BT, Philippon MJ. Evidence of validity for the hip outcome score. Arthroscopy 2006;22(12):1304–11.

11. Mohtadi NGH, Griffin DR, Pedersen ME, et al. Quality-of-life outcome measure for young, active patients. Arthroscopy 2012;28(5):595–610.

12. Griffin DR, Parsons N, Mohtadi NGH, et al. A short version of the international hip outcome tool (iHOT-12) for use in routine clinical practice. Arthroscopy 2012;28(5):611–8.

13. Thorborg K, Hölmich P, Christensen R, et al. The Copenhagen hip and groin outcome score (HAGOS): development and validation according to the COSMIN checklist. Br J Sports Med 2011;45(6):478–91.

14. Mokkink LB, Terwee CB, Patrick DL, et al. The COSMIN checklist for assessing the methodological quality of studies on measurement properties of health status measurement instruments: an international Delphi study. Qual Life Res 2010;19(4):539–49.

15. Leigh Brown AP, Kennedy ADM, Grant AM, et al. The development and validation of the Edinburgh Knee Function Scale: a simple tool for outcome measurement in non-surgical patients. Knee 1999;6(2):115–23.

16. Stratford P, Heuff J. The validation of outcome measures in patients fulfilling the clinical diagnostic criteria of chondromalacia patellae. Halifax (Canada): Annual Congress of the Canadian Physiotherapy Association; 1982.

17. Chesworth BM, Culham EG, Tata GE, et al. Validation of outcome measures in patients with patellofemoral syndrome. J Orthop Sports Phys Ther 1989;10(8):302–8.

18. Irrgang JJ, Anderson AF, Boland AL, et al. Development and validation of the international knee documentation committee subjective knee form. Am J Sports Med 2001;29(5):600–13.

19. Collins NJ, Misra D, Felson DT, et al. Measures of Knee Function: International Knee Documentation Committee (IKDC) Subjective Knee Evaluation Form, Knee Injury and Osteoarthritis Outcome Score (KOOS), Knee Injury and Osteoarthritis Outcome Score Physical Function Short Form (KOOS-PS), Knee Outcome Survey Activities of Daily Living Scale (KOS-ADL), Lysholm Knee Scoring Scale,

Oxford Knee Score (OKS), Western Ontario and McMaster Universities Osteoarthritis Index (WOMAC), Activity Rating Scale (ARS), and Tegner Activity Score (TAS). Arthritis Care Res 2011;63:S208–28.

20. Roos EM, Roos HP, Lohmander LS, et al. Knee injury and osteoarthritis outcome score (KOOS)—development of a self-administered outcome measure. J Orthop Sports Phys Ther 1998;28(2):88–96.

21. Irrgang JJ, Snyder-Mackler L, Wainner RS, et al. Development of a patient-reported measure of function of the knee. J Bone Joint Surg Am 1998; 80(8):1132–45. Available at: http://www.ncbi.nlm.nih.gov/entrez/query.fcgi?cmd=Retrieve&db=PubMed&dopt=Citation&list_uids=9730122.

22. Garratt AM, Brealey S, Robling M, et al. Development of the knee quality of life (KQoL-26) 26-item questionnaire: data quality, reliability, validity and responsiveness. Health Qual Life Outcomes 2008;6(1):48.

23. Thomee R, Wahrborg P, Borjesson M, et al. A new instrument for measuring self-efficacy in patients with an anterior cruciate ligament injury. Scand J Med Sci Sports 2006;16:181–7.

24. Bandura A. Self-efficacy: toward a unifying theory of behavioral change. Psychol Rev 1999;84(2):285–98.

25. Kujala UM, Jaakkola LH, Koskinen SK, et al. Scoring of patellofemoral disorders. Arthroscopy 1993;9(2):159–63.

26. Lysholm J, Gillquist J. Evaluation of knee ligament surgery results with special emphasis on use of a scoring scale. Am J Sports Med 1982;10(3):150–4.

27. Marx RG, Stump TJ, Jones EC, et al. Development and evaluation of an activity rating scale for disorders of the knee. Am J Sports Med 2001;29(2):213–8.

28. Tegner Y, Lysholm J. Rating systems in the evaluation of knee ligament injuries. Clin Orthop Relat Res 1985;198:43–9.

29. Marx RG, Jones EC, Allen AA, et al. Reliability, validity, and responsiveness of four knee outcome scales for athletic patients. J Bone Joint Surg Am 2001; 83-A(10):1459–69.

30. Fabricant PD, Robles A, Downey-Zayas T, et al. Development and validation of a pediatric sports activity rating scale. Am J Sports Med 2013;41(10): 2421–9.

31. Laprade JA, Culham EG. A self-administered pain severity scale for patellofemoral pain syndrome. Clin Rehabil 2002;16(7):780–8.

32. Mohtadi N. Development and validation of the quality of life outcome measure (questionnaire) for chronic anterior cruciate ligament deficiency. Am J Sports Med 1998;26(3):350–7. Available at: http://www.embase.com/search/results?subaction=viewrecord&from=export&id=L28248722%0Ahttp://resolver.ebscohost.com/openurl?custid=s3733374&authtype=ip&&sid=EMBASE&issn=03635465&id=doi:&atitle=Development+and+validation+of+the+quality+of+life+outcome+measu.

33. Kirkley A, Griffin S, Whelan D. The development and validation of a quality of life-measurement tool for patients with meniscal pathology: the Western Ontario Meniscal Evaluation Tool (WOMET). Clin J Sport Med 2007;17(5): 349–56.

34. Roach KE, Budiman-Mak E, Songsiridej N, et al. Development of a shoulder pain and disability index. Arthritis Care Res 1991;4(4):143–9.

35. Kirkley A, Alvarez C, Griffin S. The development and evaluation of a disease-specific quality-of-life questionnaire for disorders of the rotator cuff: the Western Ontario rotator cuff index. Clin J Sport Med 2003;13(2):84–92.

36. Richards RR, An K-N, Bigliani LU, et al. A standardized method for the assessment of shoulder function. J Shoulder Elbow Surg 1994;3(6):347–52.
37. Tashjian RZ, Hung M, Keener JD, et al. Determining the minimal clinically important difference for the American Shoulder and Elbow Surgeons score, Simple Shoulder Test, and visual analog scale (VAS) measuring pain after shoulder arthroplasty. J Shoulder Elbow Surg 2017;26(1):144–8.
38. Hudak PL, Amadio PC, Bombardier C. Development of an upper extremity outcome measure: the DASH (disabilities of the arm, shoulder and hand) [corrected]. The Upper Extremity Collaborative Group (UECG). Am J Ind Med 1996;29:602–8.
39. Beaton DE, Wright JG, Katz JN. QuickDASH: comparison of three item-reduction approaches. J Bone Joint Surg 2005;87-A(5):1038–46.
40. Lippitt SB, Harryman DT, Matsen FA. A practical tool for evaluating function: the simple shoulder test. In: The shoulder: a balance of mobility and stability. Rosemont (IL): American Academy of Orthopaedic Surgeons; 1993. p. 501–18.
41. Kirkley A, Griffin S, McLintock H, et al. The development and evaluation of a disease-specific quality of life measurement tool for shoulder instability. The Western Ontario Shoulder Instability Index (WOSI). Am J Sports Med 1998;26(6):764–72.
42. Lo IKY, Griffin S, Kirkley A. The development of a disease-specific quality of life measurement tool for osteoarthritis of the shoulder: the Western Ontario Osteoarthritis of the Shoulder (WOOS) index. Osteoarthr Cartil 2001;9(8):771–8.
43. Hollinshead RM, Mohtadi NGH, Vande Guchte RA, et al. Two 6-year follow-up studies of large and massive rotator cuff tears: comparison of outcome measures. J Shoulder Elbow Surg 2000;9(5):373–9.
44. Simonian PT, Sussmann PS, Wickiewicz TL, et al. Popliteomeniscal fasciculi and the unstable lateral meniscus: clinical correlation and magnetic resonance diagnosis. Arthroscopy 1997;13(5):590–6.
45. Dawson J, Fitzpatrick R, Carr A. Questionnaire on the perception of patients about shoulder surgery. J Bone Joint Surg Br 1996;78(4):593–600.
46. Williams GN, Gangel TJ, Arciero RA, et al. Comparison of the single assessment numeric evaluation method and two shoulder rating scales. Outcomes measures after shoulder surgery. Am J Sports Med 1999;27(2):214–21.
47. Brophy RH, Beauvais RL, Jones EC, et al. Measurement of shoulder activity level. Clin Orthop Relat Res 2005;439:101–8.
48. Dawson J, Doll H, Boller I, et al. The development and validation of a patient-reported questionnaire to assess outcomes of elbow surgery. J Bone Joint Surg Br 2008;90-B(4):466–73.
49. MacDermid JC. Outcome evaluation in patients with elbow pathology: issues in instrument development and evaluation. J Hand Ther 2001;14(2):105–14.
50. Papuga MO, Beck CA, Kates SL, et al. Validation of GAITRite and PROMIS as high-throughput physical function outcome measures following ACL reconstruction. J Orthop Res 2014. https://doi.org/10.1002/jor.22591.
51. Smith MV, Klein SE, Clohisy JC, et al. Lower extremity-specific measures of disability and outcomes in orthopaedic surgery. J Bone Joint Surg Am 2012; 94(5):468–77.
52. Bennell K, Bartam S, Crossley K, et al. Outcome measures in patellofemoral pain syndrome: test retest reliability and inter-relationships. Phys Ther Sport 2000;1(2): 32–41.
53. Crossley KM, Bennell KL, Cowan SM, et al. Analysis of outcome measures for persons with patellofemoral pain: which are reliable and valid? Arch Phys Med Rehabil 2004;85(5):815–22.

54. Wylie JD, Beckmann JT, Granger E, et al. Functional outcomes assessment in shoulder surgery. World J Orthop 2014;5(5):623–33.
55. Smith MV, Klein SE, Clohisy JC, et al. Upper extremity-specific measures of disability and outcomes in orthopaedic surgery. J Bone Joint Surg Am 2012; 94(5):468–77.
56. Vincent JI, MacDermid JC, King GJW, et al. Validity and sensitivity to change of patient-reported pain and disability measures for elbow pathologies. J Orthop Sports Phys Ther 2013;43(4):263–74.

Administrative Databases in Sports Medicine Research

David Wasserstein, MD, MSc, MPH, FRCSC[a,*], Ujash Sheth, MD, MSc[b]

KEYWORDS

- Administrative database • Cohort study • Epidemiology • Incidence rate
- Sports medicine

KEY POINTS

- The use of administrative databases to investigate clinical outcomes is gaining popularity within the sports medicine literature.
- Administrative databases can be broadly categorized into (1) claims-based data and (2) clinical registry–type data.
- They have improved the ability to monitor trends in practice, plan service delivery across health care systems, and detect rare complications after a procedure.
- Understanding the limitations and potential methodological issues inherent to using administrative data mitigates the risk of arriving at erroneous conclusions.

INTRODUCTION

Administrative databases are large repositories of data maintained by hospitals, health maintenance, or insurance organizations and are intended to monitor health care utilization.[1] Administrative data typically consist of billing, organizational, or system-level patient care data. Although administrative databases were not designed for observational research, the data typically allow for the investigation of regional trends, health care utilization, and outcomes of surgical intervention.[2] With the growing use of large administrative databases within the orthopedic literature, prospective researchers and consumers of this research must understand a database's characteristics, because this informs appropriate research questions and dictates the internal and external validity of the data.[3]

By their nature, all databases comprise retrospectively collected data and are unable to report clinically meaningful information in real time. The lag time between a patient encounter with a health care organization, system, or worker (eg, physician)

Disclosure Statement: The authors have nothing to disclose.
[a] Division of Orthopaedic Surgery, Sunnybrook Health Sciences Centre, University of Toronto, MG323 – 2075 Bayview Avenue, Toronto, Ontario M4N 3M5, Canada; [b] Division of Orthopaedic Surgery, University of Toronto, MG323 – 2075 Bayview Avenue, Toronto, Ontario M4N 3M5, Canada
* Corresponding author.
E-mail address: david.wasserstein@sunnybrook.ca

Clin Sports Med 37 (2018) 483–494
https://doi.org/10.1016/j.csm.2018.03.002
0278-5919/18/© 2018 Elsevier Inc. All rights reserved.

sportsmed.theclinics.com

and when the data produced from that encounter are available for analysis is occupied by data recording, verification, and cleaning. Common data categories include patient demographics, patient comorbidities, procedural information, diagnostic coding, and costs. The degree of detail and comprehensiveness is variable between data sets and, therefore, dictates the bias inherent to the study results.

Administrative databases are often confused with registries, which similarly are often confused with prospective cohorts. It is important to understand the distinction and nuances between these study types, because the granularity of data on a patient or a specific procedure/intervention level varies. Clinical registries contain large amounts of data on patient outcomes based on specific diagnoses or after common procedures (eg, hip or knee arthroplasties) with the goal of using the data to improve patient safety and health care quality.[2,4] A registry can reflect population-level outcomes when participation and completion rates are high. In sports medicine, registries for ligament reconstruction have recently been introduced,[5,6] providing information on survival (ie, time to revision) of the index operation.

Cohorts and administrative databases in some ways fit on the opposite ends of the observational study spectrum. Prospective cohorts are smaller but contain more detailed information, including patient-reported outcome measures (PROMs), which make them a valuable tool to understand who benefits most from a certain treatment. Administrative databases, however, are much larger and contain information on numerous procedures/interventions, but the outcomes available are typically binary (ie, Has an event occurred: yes or no?). Therefore, administrative databases are often best suited to evaluate complications of interventions, practice patterns, and incidence of disease. **Table 1** outlines some of the basic conceptual differences between registries, cohorts, and administrative databases.

This review focuses on administrative databases used in sports medicine research to better elucidate the types or categories of administrative data, their advantages and limitations, and some novel study designs that are possible.

TYPES OF DATABASES

One proposed classification of administrative databases is differentiating between 2 broad categories: claims-based data[2] and clinical registry–type data.[4] This differentiation can help identify what type of information is available for study. Most covariates (ie, explanatory variables) and outcomes that can be examined in administrative databases are binary—yes/no; however, some data may be continuous (eg, age

Table 1
A comparison of clinical registries, large cohorts, and administrative databases

	Registry	Cohort	Admin Database
Sample size (N)	1000s+	100s–1000s	1000s+
Number of interventions	Usually <5	Usually <5	No limit
Formulated for outcomes research?	Yes	Yes	No
PROM included	Variable	Yes	No
Radiographic data included	Variable	Yes	Variable
Generalizability	High	Based on design (no. of centers) and size	High
Follow-up	Excellent (if mandated)	Variable	Variable

and costs/reimbursements). There is no standard for procedural or diagnostic codes used between administrative databases, although there are some common patterns. Common procedural coding systems include the American Medical Association *Current Procedural Terminology (CPT)* or variants thereof, and the *International Classification of Diseases (ICD)* for diagnostic coding. Regional adaptations are common, and in general new or updated versions are more robust (eg, *ICD, Tenth Revision [ICD-10]* vs *ICD, Ninth Revision [ICD-9]*).

Claims-Based

There are 2 claims-based databases used in sports medicine research—Medicare and PearlDiver.

Medicare

The Medicare database is one of the largest and most complete administrative databases for individuals over the age of 65. As of 2012, there were more than 45 million people enrolled in Medicare.[2] It is somewhat limited, however, for research on sports medicine or soft tissue injuries, because the program provides insurance for people age 65 years and older and only a small number of patients younger than 65 who have certain disabilities. In addition, some patients over the age of 65 may engage the US health care system using their private insurance over Medicare and, therefore, not all interactions with the health care system in those greater than 65 years of age are captured. Available data include *ICD-9* and *ICD-10* diagnostic coding, billing information (via *CPT* coding), and select pharmaceutical information.

Medicare databases have been used within the sports medicine literature to examine risks of infection after hip[7] and elbow arthroscopy[8] and to compare costs in rotator cuff repair.[9]

PearlDiver

PearlDiver is a health analytics company that maintains a physician claims database that comprises both large private insurer and public Medicare claims data dating back to 2007.[2] The database contains *CPT* and *ICD* coding and is available for research purposes for an annual subscription fee. There has been a significant increase in the publication of orthopedic studies using the PearlDiver database. Previous studies have evaluated practice patterns for common orthopedic conditions, whereas others have examined early complication rates, such as revision or infection. Recent publications have reported on surgical trends in the knee,[10] hip,[11] elbow,[12] ankle,[13] and shoulder.[14] Due to concerns regarding loss or change of insurance status, most studies have focused on short-term (eg, 30-day) outcomes, because assessment of long-term outcomes may introduce significant bias with changing coverage.

Health Systems/Organizations

Health systems/organization databases may also contain billing/claims data but are designed from the perspective of examining regional/geographic health system use. Many European countries have administrative databases that track basic procedural and diagnostic codes from all inpatient and outpatient hospital encounters.

Statewide Planning and Research Cooperative System Database

The Statewide Planning and Research Cooperative System (SPARCS) database is an administrative database that collects New York State hospital data and has been used in several sports medicine studies.[15–17] The SPARCS database evolved from a pure hospital discharge database to one that collects information from all inpatient and outpatient encounters, including procedural and diagnostic coding, across all insurance types. It has been used to investigate the effects of legislative changes on practice,[15] examine reoperation and other similar outcomes after common orthopedic procedures,[18] and examine patterns of health care utilization in New York State or in comparison to other jurisdictions.[16,17,19]

Linked/Complex Databases

There are a few examples of administrative databases that have features of both regional/systems and claims databases. These databases are often more mature and run by dedicated research organizations that create unique subcohorts via anonymous patient identification numbers to allow complex database linkages while maintaining privacy. Although the data from linked databases can be richer, understanding their nuances is still important.

Kaiser Permanente

Kaiser Permanente (KP) is a large private insurer based out of California that gathers not only administrative database types of information (eg, demographic data and diagnostic and procedural coding) but also prospective data (eg, patient-reported outcomes and implants used) on patients treated within their network through a dedicated research institution. Reporting is mandatory and patients are provided with a unique anonymized identification number. The database has its limitations, however, because the population consists of only those individuals with KP coverage. Irrespective of its shortcomings, it remains an excellent source for high-quality integrated data. There have been more than 20 publications in sports medicine using KP data, most of which have come from the California region.[20–24]

Institute for Clinical Evaluative Sciences

The Institute for Clinical Evaluative Sciences (ICES) is an independent, nonprofit, health services research organization that provides secure access to linked deidentified health care databases in the province of Ontario, Canada. Linkages have been created between various health care databases, including population statistics, claims data, inpatient and outpatient hospital encounters, public health surveys, and trauma registries, to name a few. In the province of Ontario, the Ontario Health Insurance Plan (OHIP) acts as a single-payer, universal health plan for its citizens, thereby providing coverage for more than 95% of physician services for a population of approximately 13.5 million people.[25] The physician fee codes contained in the OHIP billing database have been found to have excellent reliability in numerous validation studies.[25] These databases provide no information on patient-reported outcomes, and reporting of specific procedure-related details, however, such as laterality, can vary.

EVALUATING ADMINISTRATIVE DATABASE RESEARCH
Overview

There are many validated tools for a structured approach to reviewing observational cohort studies, such as Strengthening the Reporting of Observational Studies in Epidemiology (STROBE)[26] and Quality in Prognostic Studies.[27] The REporting of studies Conducted using Observational Routinely-collected health Data (RECORD)[28] tool is a 13-item checklist that was developed as an extension to STROBE.[29] The intent of the RECORD checklist is to facilitate structured peer review of studies conducted using routinely collected health data, such as administrative database and registry studies. The authors have adapted 3 key principles that are necessary for a basic evaluation by anyone appraising this literature.

Principle 1: understand the population

The source population is the population the researcher intends to make inferences on. The database population is contained within the source population and represented by the individuals captured in the database. The study population is the cohort of patients within the database population who have been identified based on combinations of codes. The reader should always consider whether the study population sufficiently represents the source population (ie, external validity or generalizability).

Most administrative databases in sports medicine are derived from insurance plans, in other words, the population of persons with that type of insurance, whether it is private (eg, KP or PearlDiver) or public (eg, OHIP or Medicare). Other database populations comprise regional hospital–level data (eg, SPARCS or ICES/Ontario). Depending on the study question, neither database population may encompass the entire geographic or source population affected.

Consider a study examining shoulder instability on a national or state/provincial level. If a researcher wants to examine patterns or risk factors for dislocation, a hospital-level–only study might not capture patients who went to walk-in clinics after autoreduction or who were reduced on a playing field. A database with combined hospital and claims data might capture more patients depending on how much of the population was covered by the insurance type. In contrast, if a researcher wanted to study early reoperation after shoulder instability repair, a claims database would only identify a subset of persons in that region with that type of insurance and limit the generalizability of the conclusions to the type of patients covered. In contrast, in this scenario, a registry-type database that contained all hospital/day surgery interactions may provide more representative data because the procedures must take place in those locations.

Principle 2: evaluate the study population definition

The study population is otherwise known as the index population—the group of patients within the database who had the initial event of interest (eg, shoulder dislocation or anterior cruciate ligament reconstruction [ACLR]). A researcher does not need to be a coding expert to assess the quality of coding used in the study. First, an article must include a list of the codes used and algorithms instituted by the investigators. Are these codes too generic or are they specific enough to capture the study population as it was defined? For example, some coding may not specify which ligament of the knee was injured—can it reliably be inferred that this is an anterior cruciate ligament (ACL) study?

More sophisticated administrative data methodology use 1 or both of the following features:

1. Algorithms of codes from multiple sources
2. Code validation (discussed later)

Principle 3: review the limitations of the study

Administrative databases were not created or collected to answer clinical questions. The main limitations of these data sets include misclassification bias, the presence of unmeasured confounding variables, missing data, and the changing eligibility of study patients over time.

Basics of Study Design

The stalwart of study design and statistical analysis relevant to administrative databases is retrospective cohort studies and regression analysis. Cohort studies are observational studies that track greater than or equal to 2 groups forward from an exposure to an outcome and are either prospective or retrospective.[30] Administrative database cohort studies can be used to examine the incidence (ie, patterns at one time or over time) and natural history of common conditions. Whether univariate or multivariate regression analysis is possible depends on the degrees of freedom among covariates and the number of observed outcomes.

One of the most common uses for administrative databases is to provide information on surgical practice patterns over time and by jurisdiction. These data are useful for health services research and fiscal planning. For example, the authors performed a study of primary ACLR in Ontario, Canada,[31] that demonstrated a change in practice from predominantly inpatient to predominantly outpatient procedures during the 1990s and early 2000s. These data were helpful in establishing benchmarks for cost and for demonstrating to administrators that outpatient surgery was the standard of care. In the era of bundled payments and episodes of care, the value provided by these types of data will only increase.

A case-control study is defined as a study where the case is defined first, often a rare outcome or occurrence, and then matched to multiple controls (eg, 3:1 or more) of a similar exposure but that did not experience the outcome. These studies are by definition retrospective and can be done nested within a cohort.[32] Cases and controls are compared to identify factors that differed and may be associated with (but not cause) the outcome. For example, Spragg and colleagues[20] identified cases of failed hamstring tendon autograft ACLR first and then matched these individuals to similar persons with a nonrevised autograft hamstring ACLR to examine the association of graft diameter on failure.

Other cohort variants are amenable to administrative database research. A matched cohort study compares the outcome of 2 similar subcohorts who have undergone a similar exposure. For example, the authors' group performed a matched cohort study of meniscal repair with and without ACLR in patients of similar age, gender, and co-morbidity.[33] Although these designs cannot account for every difference between patients, the more characteristics that are matched, the more similar the cohorts will become. The resulting statistics in matched cohort studies are simpler to design and interpret (eg, McNemar test or paired t test) compared with complex regression analysis.

Other novel study designs have also been introduced into administrative database research. The propensity score matching design is worth discussion,[34,35] although it has not yet made its way into sports medicine administrative database research. In simple terms, propensity score matching is a tool for observational research that attempts to reduce bias by accounting for covariates that predict receiving the treatment.[36] A simple example might be age and likelihood of receiving ACLR after a tear or in tearing a reconstructed ACL. Propensity score matching in some ways reduces the bias of treatment decisions between groups, much like a randomized controlled trial (RCT). It is not as powerful, however, as an RCT, because an RCT can account for both known and unknown confounders through the process of randomization, whereas propensity score matching only accounts for known confounders.[36]

Case study: acute Achilles tendon ruptures

Administrative data sets have been used to examine how treatment approaches have evolved on a population level. For example, recent RCT evidence has emerged in the orthopedic literature that suggests a stronger role for nonoperative management in acute Achilles tendon ruptures.[37] Accordingly, various research groups have examined operative rates for acute repair and in some jurisdictions demonstrated an expected decrease in operative management (Canada and Europe[38–40]). In contrast, administrative database studies found little change in surgical rates in the public US Medicare database[41] and a small increase in operative rate among privately insured US patients over a similar time period[42] (**Table 2**). Four of the studies also examined the population incidence of acute Achilles tendon rupture rate over time, and all demonstrated an increase.

There is a lot of value in this conglomerate of data, which highlights some of the main practical utilities of administrative database research. First, the incidence of Achilles tendon rupture seems to be increasing globally. This evidence is strong enough on its own to warrant further research into potential causes and concurrently to begin conceptualizing injury prevention methods, including public education. Second, there are different practice patterns around the world. These findings suggest a need to understand why and perhaps increase knowledge translation and dissemination to providers. There are some limitations, however, of drawing conclusions from practice pattern data: (1) the reason for regional differences cannot be inferred (ie, why patterns have changed in some areas and not others); (2) the data collected may not be similar enough to compare raw numbers; and (3) the best treatment choice for an individual patient's needs cannot be deduced solely from population-based research or randomized trials.

Learning point 1: identify the denominator

Administrative data are good at providing population-level epidemiologic data (ie, rates or incidence of injury and treatment). When examining **Table 2**, however, it is apparent that the rate of surgical repair is not presented in a uniform manner among different studies, thus limiting direct comparison of these numbers. As a result, it must always be considered what the denominator is.

Is the denominator number of operative cases per population? A Finnish study[38] presented operative rates as a function of the general population (in person-years). Data on nonoperatively treated patients were not presented.

Is the denominator number of operative cases per total number of acute Achilles tendon ruptures? If so, how accurate or encompassing are the data on acute tendon ruptures? How much of the population does the database service (ie, source

Table 2
Administrative database studies examining treatment patterns for acute Achilles tendon rupture

Jurisdiction	Type of Insurance	Sample Size	Years	Trend in Surgical Management (% operative or incidence)
Ontario (Canada)[39]	Public	27,607	2003–2013	20% → 9%
Finland[38]	Public	15,252 (surgical pts only)	1987–2011	1987: 11.1/100,000 person-years 2008: 35.5/100,000 person-years 2011: 20.5/100,000 person-years[a]
Sweden[40]	Public	27,702	2001–2012	43% → 28% (men) 34% → 22% (women)
United States[42]	Private	12,570	2007–2011	58% → 62%
United States[41]	Public (Medicare)	14,127	2005–2011	Raw data not given; rates "unchanged" at ~30%

[a] Incidence density rate of surgical repair for men only (rates of women lower).

population and database population)? These patients may present and be treated in multiple settings (emergency department, walk-in clinic, private office, and so forth), so if the denominator is the total number of acute ruptures, that may differ based on the type of database. Swedish[40] and Canadian[39] studies examined patients who presented as either inpatient or outpatient to a hospital. Both databases also included either public/private mix (Sweden) or all public (Canada) insurance coverage in those jurisdictions, meaning they were more likely to capture all acute ruptures in the source population. In contrast, databases of only private insurance would capture a subset of patients with potential regional, gender, age, and socioeconomic differences and, therefore, may not be representative of the source population. If a researcher believes that any of these factors (or covariates) influenced the likelihood of sustaining an Achilles tendon rupture (eg, age and gender are known confounders) or in the likelihood of undergoing repair, then far greater bias may be introduced into the denominator.

Learning point 2: trends cannot imply causality
Trends observed in administrative database study designs do not imply causality, but they can be hypothesis generating and therefore form the basis of more detailed investigation.

Additional Pearls and Pitfalls

Tracking patients in follow-up
Because most administrative databases provide binary answers to outcomes of clinical interest, the ability to obtain high-quality and less biased data on those outcomes requires good data capture in follow-up. Some databases capture only information for a single admission, and, because patients are not identifiable (usually due to privacy issues), they are lost to follow-up once discharged. The National Trauma Data Bank is an example of such a database. Events that take place during admission are well captured, but those that occur subsequently, such as during readmission or reoperation/revision, are not.[4] A study from these databases tell a limited story.

Regional databases may have similar limitations if they are designed from an institutional rather than individual perspective. Persons who move out of the catchment zone,[18] lose insurance status, or die may not be captured if they are not tracked. The potential for introducing loss to follow-up bias increases for outcomes that are sought far from the index event. An example might be looking for conversion of rotator cuff repairs to reverse total shoulder arthroplasty. Such a study could be reliably performed in a database that is able to track causes of loss to follow-up from death, insurance status change, or emigration, known as competing risks, and special types of similarly named regression analysis may be performed.[43]

Data quality and completeness
It is generally recommended that only databases that have had previous code validation performed and published, or ones where the investigators perform a code validation on their own, be used for administrative database research. Code validation studies essentially confirm the accuracy of a coding algorithm by comparing codes in the entire cohort (uncommon) or a random subset (more common) of the study to patient charts. This allows the calculation of code sensitivity and positive predictive value.[25]

There are no specific published code validation studies in sports medicine. Many reasons may account for this, including a lack of familiarity of the process by researchers, the more recent introduction of these types of studies to the field, and the cost and time associated with performing them. Some administrative databases used commonly in sports medicine undergo regular unpublished internal validation (eg, PearlDiver), non–peer-reviewed published validation,[25] or validation in other fields.

The type of database may also influence the accuracy of the available data and accordingly the strength of conclusions from any one study. For example, discordances for complications have been observed between claims-based data and chart-abstracted data among similar cohorts.[44]

Spurious associations and conclusions

Because most databases produce large data sets, there are often many questions that can be asked. Although this is an advantage in some settings, such as when powering regression analyses for infrequent outcomes, it may lead to statistically significant associations that lack clinical plausibility. Furthermore, it may lead to type 1 errors, and consultation with a statistician is recommended to determine whether multiple comparison corrections of a P value are indicated.

For example, a recent study examining the effect of concomitant biceps tenodesis on reoperation rates after arthroscopic rotator cuff repair utilized a large private-payer database.[14] The investigators found a statistically significantly higher rate of reoperation in those individuals who underwent concomitant biceps tenodesis and of postoperative urinary tract infection in those who did not have a tenodesis. The latter association obviously lacks plausibility and clinical relevance.

NOVEL STUDY DESIGNS AND FUTURE DIRECTIONS

Some researchers have endeavored to perform database linkage studies between jurisdictions. These can be a challenge for numerous reasons, including privacy issues (anonymized data are required) and whether the coding utilized in each database is similar. If successful, however, they offer an opportunity to examine trends in treatment patterns over time between jurisdictions or even between types of health care systems (public, private, and mixed).

In 1 study,[17] the incidence of repair for superior labral tears from anterior to posterior (SLAPs) was queried among administrative databases in New York State, California, and the American Board of Orthopaedic Surgery (ABOS) database. The latter is a database of case mix information on surgeons in their first 2 years of practice as they head to step 2 board certification in the United States. They demonstrated a dramatic rise in SLAP repairs among statewide databases from the early to late 2000s; no such trend was observed in the ABOS database. The results suggest there was a difference in general practice compared with those new in practice but also that practice patterns may be different when surgical cases are monitored (ie, during the first 2 years of practice). The investigators opined that they expected the incidence of SLAP repairs to decrease as knowledge of indications for successful repair have narrowed. These types of data are important because they highlight the need for further knowledge translation and/or open reporting of procedures.

SUMMARY

During the past decade, there has been a dramatic increase in the publication of orthopedic sports medicine studies using large health administrative databases. The use of big data[45] has improved the ability to monitor trends in practice, plan service delivery across health care systems, and detect rare adverse events, such as complications after a procedure.[46] Despite the growing appeal of having large data sets readily available for analysis, investigators must remember that these databases were never designed to answer clinical questions, thereby creating potential methodological issues, many of which are touched on in this article. Therefore, recognizing these limitations and adhering to well-established principles of scientific rigor when navigating through these studies will help avoid propagating spurious conclusions.

REFERENCES

1. Gavrielov-Yusim N, Friger M. Use of administrative medical databases in population-based research. J Epidemiol Community Health 2014;68(3):283–7.
2. Pugely AJ, Martin CT, Harwood J, et al. Database and registry research in orthopaedic surgery: part 1: claims-based data. J Bone Joint Surg Am 2015;97(15): 1278–87.
3. Weinreb JH, Yoshida R, Cote MP, et al. A review of databases used in orthopaedic surgery research and an analysis of database use in arthroscopy: the journal of arthroscopic and related surgery. Arthroscopy 2017;33(1):225–31.
4. Pugely AJ, Martin CT, Harwood J, et al. Database and registry research in orthopaedic surgery: part 2: clinical registry data. J Bone Joint Surg Am 2015;97(21): 1799–808.
5. Granan LP, Bahr R, Steindal K, et al. Development of a national cruciate ligament surgery registry: the Norwegian National Knee Ligament Registry. Am J Sports Med 2008;36(2):308–15.
6. Granan LP, Forssblad M, Lind M, et al. The Scandinavian ACL registries 2004-2007: baseline epidemiology. Acta Orthop 2009;80(5):563–7.
7. Wang D, Camp CL, Ranawat AS, et al. The timing of hip arthroscopy after intra-articular hip injection affects postoperative infection risk. Arthroscopy 2017; 33(11):1988–94. e1981.
8. Camp CL, Cancienne JM, Degen RM, et al. Factors that increase the risk of infection after elbow arthroscopy: analysis of patient demographics, medical comorbidities, and steroid injections in 2,704 medicare patients. Arthroscopy 2017; 33(6):1175–9.
9. Narvy SJ, Didinger TC, Lehoang D, et al. Direct cost analysis of outpatient arthroscopic rotator cuff repair in medicare and non-medicare populations. Orthop J Sports Med 2016;4(10). 2325967116668829.
10. Arshi A, Cohen JR, Wang JC, et al. Operative management of patellar instability in the United States: an evaluation of national practice patterns, surgical trends, and complications. Orthop J Sports Med 2016;4(8). 2325967116662873.
11. Truntzer JN, Hoppe DJ, Shapiro LM, et al. Complication rates for hip arthroscopy are underestimated: a population-based study. Arthroscopy 2017;33(6): 1194–201.
12. Wang D, Joshi NB, Petrigliano FA, et al. Trends associated with distal biceps tendon repair in the United States, 2007 to 2011. J Shoulder Elbow Surg 2016; 25(4):676–80.
13. Yasui Y, Murawski CD, Wollstein A, et al. Reoperation rates following ankle ligament procedures performed with and without concomitant arthroscopic procedures. Knee Surg Sports Traumatol Arthrosc 2017;25(6):1908–15.
14. Erickson BJ, Basques BA, Griffin JW, et al. The effect of concomitant biceps tenodesis on reoperation rates after rotator cuff repair: a review of a large private-payer database from 2007 to 2014. Arthroscopy 2017;33(7):1301–7.e1.
15. Baker DR, Kulick ER, Boehme AK, et al. Effects of the New York State Concussion Management and Awareness Act ("Lystedt Law") on concussion-related

emergency health care utilization among adolescents, 2005-2015. Am J Sports Med 2018;46(2):396–401.

16. Degen RM, Bernard JA, Pan TJ, et al. Hip arthroscopy utilization and associated complications: a population-based analysis. J Hip Preserv Surg 2017;4(3):240–9.

17. Vogel LA, Moen TC, Macaulay AA, et al. Superior labrum anterior-to-posterior repair incidence: a longitudinal investigation of community and academic databases. J Shoulder Elbow Surg 2014;23(6):e119–26.

18. Lyman S, Koulouvaris P, Sherman S, et al. Epidemiology of anterior cruciate ligament reconstruction: trends, readmissions, and subsequent knee surgery. J Bone Joint Surg Am 2009;91(10):2321–8.

19. Ensor KL, Kwon YW, Dibeneditto MR, et al. The rising incidence of rotator cuff repairs. J Shoulder Elbow Surg 2013;22(12):1628–32.

20. Spragg L, Chen J, Mirzayan R, et al. The effect of autologous hamstring graft diameter on the likelihood for revision of anterior cruciate ligament reconstruction. Am J Sports Med 2016;44(6):1475–81.

21. Inacio MC, Paxton EW, Maletis GB, et al. Patient and surgeon characteristics associated with primary anterior cruciate ligament reconstruction graft selection. Am J Sports Med 2012;40(2):339–45.

22. Inacio MC, Cafri G, Funahashi TT, et al. Type and frequency of healthcare encounters can predict poor surgical outcomes in anterior cruciate ligament reconstruction patients. Int J Med Inform 2016;90:32–9.

23. Maletis GB, Inacio MC, Funahashi TT. Risk factors associated with revision and contralateral anterior cruciate ligament reconstructions in the kaiser permanente ACLR registry. Am J Sports Med 2015;43(3):641–7.

24. Maletis GB, Chen J, Inacio MC, et al. Age-related risk factors for revision anterior cruciate ligament reconstruction: a cohort study of 21,304 patients from the kaiser permanente anterior cruciate ligament registry. Am J Sports Med 2016;44(2):331–6.

25. Williams JI, Young W. A summary of studies on the quality of health care administrative databases in canada. In: Goel V, Williams JI, Anderson GM, et al, editors. Patterns of health care in ontario. 2nd edition. Ottawa: Canadian Medical Association; 1996.

26. Vandenbroucke JP, von Elm E, Altman DG, et al. Strengthening the reporting of observational studies in epidemiology (STROBE): explanation and elaboration. Int J Surg 2014;12(12):1500–24.

27. Hayden JA, Cote P, Bombardier C. Evaluation of the quality of prognosis studies in systematic reviews. Ann Intern Med 2006;144(6):427–37.

28. Benchimol EI, Smeeth L, Guttmann A, et al. The reporting of studies conducted using observational routinely-collected health data (RECORD) statement. PLoS Med 2015;12(10):e1001885.

29. Nicholls SG, Quach P, von Elm E, et al. The reporting of studies conducted using observational routinely-collected health data (RECORD) statement: methods for arriving at consensus and developing reporting guidelines. PLoS One 2015; 10(5):e0125620.

30. Grimes DA, Schulz KF. Cohort studies: marching towards outcomes. Lancet 2002;359(9303):341–5.

31. Wasserstein D, Khoshbin A, Dwyer T, et al. Risk factors for recurrent anterior cruciate ligament reconstruction: a population study in Ontario, Canada, with 5-year follow-up. Am J Sports Med 2013;41(9):2099–107.

32. Sedgwick P. Nested case-control studies. BMJ 2010;340:c2582.

33. Wasserstein D, Dwyer T, Gandhi R, et al. A matched-cohort population study of reoperation after meniscal repair with and without concomitant anterior cruciate ligament reconstruction. Am J Sports Med 2013;41(2):349–55.

34. Austin PC. A comparison of 12 algorithms for matching on the propensity score. Stat Med 2014;33(6):1057–69.
35. Austin PC. The use of propensity score methods with survival or time-to-event outcomes: reporting measures of effect similar to those used in randomized experiments. Stat Med 2014;33(7):1242–58.
36. Austin PC. An introduction to propensity score methods for reducing the effects of confounding in observational studies. Multivariate Behav Res 2011;46(3): 399–424.
37. Soroceanu A, Sidhwa F, Aarabi S, et al. Surgical versus nonsurgical treatment of acute Achilles tendon rupture: a meta-analysis of randomized trials. J Bone Joint Surg Am 2012;94(23):2136–43.
38. Mattila VM, Huttunen TT, Haapasalo H, et al. Declining incidence of surgery for Achilles tendon rupture follows publication of major RCTs: evidence-influenced change evident using the Finnish registry study. Br J Sports Med 2015;49(16): 1084–6.
39. Sheth U, Wasserstein D, Jenkinson R, et al. The epidemiology and trends in management of acute Achilles tendon ruptures in Ontario, Canada: a population-based study of 27 607 patients. Bone Joint J 2017;99-B(1):78–86.
40. Huttunen TT, Kannus P, Rolf C, et al. Acute Achilles tendon ruptures: incidence of injury and surgery in Sweden between 2001 and 2012. Am J Sports Med 2014; 42(10):2419–23.
41. Erickson BJ, Cvetanovich GL, Nwachukwu BU, et al. Trends in the management of Achilles tendon ruptures in the United States medicare population, 2005-2011. Orthop J Sports Med 2014;2(9). 2325967114549948.
42. Wang D, Sandlin MI, Cohen JR, et al. Operative versus nonoperative treatment of acute Achilles tendon rupture: an analysis of 12,570 patients in a large healthcare database. Foot Ankle Surg 2015;21(4):250–3.
43. Leroux T, Ogilvie-Harris D, Veillette C, et al. The epidemiology of primary anterior shoulder dislocations in patients aged 10 to 16 years. Am J Sports Med 2015; 43(9):2111–7.
44. Patterson JT, Sing D, Hansen EN, et al. The James A. Rand Young Investigator's award: administrative claims vs surgical registry: capturing outcomes in total joint arthroplasty. J Arthroplasty 2017;32(9S):S11–7.
45. Pugely AJ, Bozic KJ. Editorial commentary: rising interest in "Big Data" in arthroscopy: is the juice worth the squeeze? Arthroscopy 2017;33(1):232–3.
46. Perry DC, Parsons N, Costa ML. 'Big data' reporting guidelines: how to answer big questions, yet avoid big problems. Bone Joint J 2014;96-B(12):1575–7.

To MOON and Back
Lessons Learned and Experience Gained Along the Way

José F. Vega, MA[a,b], Kurt P. Spindler, MD[b],*

KEYWORDS

- MOON • knee • Prospective cohort • Multicenter • Outcomes ACL

KEY POINTS

- The Multicenter Orthopaedic Outcomes Network (MOON) is one of the largest prospective cohorts in orthopaedic sports medicine, with more than 4,000 anterior cruciate ligament reconstructions (ACLRs) enrolled.
- Bringing the dream of MOON to fruition took more than a decade of planning. Among many topics, this article describes the early cohort studies that ultimately paved the way for MOON.
- When working with teams of researchers, it is vital to demonstrate that the data collected by different individuals is scientifically valid. This article also reviews the agreement studies done in preparation for MOON.
- Conducting multicenter orthopaedic research requires a large and diverse team, with individuals of different backgrounds and areas of expertise including physicians, epidemiologists, biostatisticians, physical therapists, research coordinators, and many more.
- Although conducting multicenter orthopaedic research is challenging, the story of MOON provides many valuable lessons that can help those aiming to design or participate in multicenter research.

Disclosure: Research reported in this publication was supported by the National Institute of Arthritis and Musculoskeletal and Skin Diseases of the National Institutes of Health (NIH) under Award Number R01 AR053684 (K.P. Spindler). The content is solely the responsibility of the authors and does not necessarily represent the official views of the NIH. The project was also supported by the Vanderbilt Sports Medicine Research Fund (R01AR053684), which received unrestricted educational gifts from Smith & Nephew Endoscopy and DonJoy Orthopedics.

a Orthopaedics Sports Medicine, Cleveland Clinic Lerner College of Medicine, Case Western Reserve University, 5555 Transportation Boulevard, Garfield Heights, Cleveland, OH 44125, USA; b Orthopaedic Sports Medicine, Cleveland Clinic, 5555 Transportation Boulevard, Garfield Heights, Cleveland, OH 44125, USA
* Corresponding author. Orthopaedic and Rheumatologic Institute, Cleveland Clinic, Cleveland, OH, 44195.
E-mail addresses: spindlk@ccf.org; sosice@ccf.org

Clin Sports Med 37 (2018) 495–503
https://doi.org/10.1016/j.csm.2018.03.003
0278-5919/18/© 2018 Elsevier Inc. All rights reserved.

sportsmed.theclinics.com

"That's one small step for man, one giant leap for mankind."

These words were immortalized by Neil Armstrong as he stepped out of the lunar module Eagle in the summer of 1969, marking the successful culmination of the Apollo space program and the fulfillment of the late President John F. Kennedy's 1961 promise to land a man on the moon before the end of the decade. Given that only a few months had elapsed between Russian cosmonaut Yuri Gagarin's maiden voyage into space and President Kennedy's promise, some might have considered the president's goal impossible. Today, some might refer to such a promise as a BHAG – a big, hairy audacious goal – a term coined by James Collins and Jerry Porras in their 1994 book *Built to Last: Successful Habits of Visionary Companies*. It took only a mere 9 years from the first human trip into space until Armstrong and Aldrin's famous moon walk. Needless to say, there were countless hours poured into planning the Apollo 11 mission, and equally as many hurdles to overcome in order to make President Kennedy's dream a reality. Much like Apollo 11, the story of MOON is one of vision, teamwork, perseverance, and (thankfully) success. And, also like Apollo 11, MOON's (Multicenter Orthopedic Outcomes Network) story began long before its official launch, with more than a decade of thought and planning preceding the enrollment of the first study participant in 2002.

The journey to the MOON really began during one author's fellowship year at Cleveland Clinic in 1990, a full 12 years before the authors enrolled their first patient into what has now become the largest prospective anterior cruciate ligament reconstruction (ACLR) cohort with at least 80% follow-up in the world. The story starts with a much smaller prospective cohort study involving a mere 54 patients who had undergone acute (within 3 months of injury) ACLR at Cleveland Clinic during the year of that fellwoship.[1]

At the time, it was well established that knees undergoing primary ACL repair had a high failure rate by their fourth postoperative year, and it was beginning to be realized that ACL reconstruction utilizing an autograft led to a more anatomically stable knee while also reducing the incidence of subsequent meniscus tears. In addition, chronic ACL deficiency seemed to be associated with both worse outcomes and the development of post-traumatic osteoarthritis.[2–5] Additionally during this time period, a growing body of literature suggested that ACL reconstruction improved knee stability and function, at least in the short term (2 years after surgery).[6] However, what remained largely unknown and at the forefront of many orthopedic sports medicine surgeons' minds was, given the myriad of associated injuries that concomitantly occurred at the time of an ACL tear (eg, meniscus tears, articular cartilage injuries, and bone bruises), which types of injuries or treatments were predictive of clinically relevant outcomes. Furthermore, whether ACLR decreased the incidence of future post-traumatic osteoarthritis was unknown. Thus, beginning in the fall of 1990, the authors enrolled 54 patients with the goal of determining the association between bone bruises seen on MRI and meniscus and articular cartilage injuries. In addition, the authors hoped to follow this cohort for 10 years to shed some light on longer term outcomes. The authors were naïve to believe that they could determine which preoperative and intraoperative variables (specifically the presence of bone bruising and/or meniscus or articular cartilage injuries) could be used to predict long-term outcomes in such a small dataset.[1,7]

It did not take long for the authors to realize that there were likely a multitude of variables beyond intra-articular injuries that impacted both the development of post-traumatic osteoarthritis and long-term patient-reported outcomes measures (PROMs). Furthermore, with the increased utilization of ACL reconstruction rather than the traditional repair, new and important questions arose that also needed answering such as what graft to use (autograft or allograft, hamstring or bone-patellar tendon-bone [BTB]) and how to decide. Consequently, it became obvious that the authors' prospective cohort of 54 patients would not suffice to answer such complex questions.

It was on a hot summer day in 1991 that Dr. Jack Andrish (Cleveland Clinic, Cleveland, Ohio) and one of the authors found themselves on an early morning bike ride in Sun Valley, Idaho, deep in the midst of a discussion revolving around the metaphorical elephant in the room – the fact that it would likely take hundreds, if not thousands, of ACLR patients in a meticulously designed prospective cohort study to answer the myriad of multifaceted questions surrounding predictors or risk factors of ACLR outcomes and ACLR's long-term impact. Naturally, once they conceded that there would be no way around this hurdle (short of performing dozens of parallel cohort studies or randomized trials), the discussion shifted to how we could possibly enroll, in a reasonable period of time, and follow thousands of patients that undergo a procedure that, at the time, was being performed less than 90,000 times nationwide annually.[8] The answer, of course, was to collaborate between institutions and form a multicenter network.

In 1991, having finished his fellowship at Cleveland Clinic, one of the authors headed south to start his career as an assistant professor at Vanderbilt University (Nashville, TN), and, thus, the Vanderbilt Sports Medicine-Cleveland Clinic Foundation (VSM-CCF) ACLR Registry was born. Between the latter half of 1991 and 1998, that author and colleagues captured baseline demographics, PROMs (eg, Lysholm scale), the type of ACLR, and the treatment of meniscus and articular cartilage injuries. They enrolled a total of 1201 ACLR patients between 3 surgeons (Jack Andrish, Richard Parker, and one of the authors) with the aim of following these patients for 5 years. Around this time, we also developed a new relationship, this time with The Ohio State University (Dr. Christopher Kaeding), which was also assembling a similar database of its own ACLR cohort. This new partnership nearly doubled the size of the existing cohort, bringing the final number to 2286 ACLRs between 3 institutions over roughly a decade. However, there were no follow-up mechanism for these ACLR patients from whom baseline information had been captured. Given the size of this new cohort, if one could achieve reasonable follow-up, one would be able to not only observe the natural history of an ACL reconstructed knee, but also be able to perform more complex multivariable regression analyses to identify preoperative and intraoperative variables that could predict outcomes.

Unlike the authors' initial 52-patient cohort, this initial multicenter ACLR registry would require a significant investment of resources in order to achieve meaningful follow-up. As a result, the authors and colleagues applied for a Prospective Clinical Research Grant from the Orthopedic Research and Education Foundation (OREF), and, as is often the case when applying for funding, the first submission was rejected. However, the authors were successfully funded after revising their initial submission, thus providing the necessary financial resources to create a research infrastructure capable of achieving 70% to 80% follow-up of a subset (over 300 ACLRs) that was at least 5 years removed from surgery.

The goal of achieving follow-up on a large ACLR cohort spanning multiple institutions came to fruition in 2005, when the authors were able to demonstrate the feasibility of their concept and provide a small sample of the wide range of information that could be gleaned from a large, well-designed prospective cohort.[9] In total, the 3-institution ACLR registry produced 8 publications on a wide range of topics including predictors of intra-articular injuries, a comparison of intra-articular injury patterns between high school and recreational athletes, a description of common intra-articular findings in the multiligamentously injured knee, and outcomes of 2 medial meniscal repair techniques.[9–16]

What made the initial registry unique was not only its size (at the time, it was one of the largest prospectively assembled ACLR cohorts in the United States), but also its overall design. In addition to investing an incredible amount of effort into collecting outcomes, the authors also recorded a variety of preoperative and intraoperative variables. Doing so allowed the authors to perform multivariable regression modeling to identify predictors of outcomes, a novel concept to sports medicine and orthopedics at the time. Thus, with their single cohort, the authors were able to answer multiple questions simultaneously. Possibly the most unique (perhaps controversial would be more accurate) facet of the authors' initial multicenter cohort was the use of 2 PROMs that had recently been designed and validated for use in a knee surgery population – the International Knee Documentation Committee Subjective Knee Form (IKDC-SKF) and the Knee injury and Osteoarthritis Outcome Score (KOOS).[17,18]

The authors' use of the IKDC-SKF and the KOOS as primary endpoints represented a major paradigm shift in the way in which orthopedic research was conducted and critically evaluated. Consequently, the design – to use PROMs as a primary outcome without objective data to accompany it (such as radiograph measurements or arthrometer recordings) was met with considerable trepidation, which, in the fall of 2005 and spring of 2006, played out in a public way.[19,20] Nevertheless, the methodology was ultimately accepted as a scientifically valid approach to ACLR follow-up, thereby paving the way for MOON, which, at the time, was already underway but in need of additional external financial support, to be seriously considered as a concept worth federal funding.

Despite the knowledge that had been gained from the 3-center cohort, it seemed that 10 new questions arose for each question that was addressed. Again, the authors were humbled by the need for more information, and, again, had to admit that there were many additional questions that the 3-center ACLR cohort, which was designed to understand the long-term impact of intra-articular injuries and treatment sustained during ACL rupture, simply could not answer. Also complicating matters was the development of new methods for measuring outcomes, like the IKDC and the KOOS, which debuted after enrollment was completed, thereby creating a gap in the baseline dataset and rendering the authors unable to compare baseline values to those collected postoperatively. Thus, the authors knew they needed to establish a new prospective cohort that was larger and derived from more patients than the 3 institutions could provide. Answering more questions would require more data, which meant more patients, more surgeons, and more institutions.

Ultimately, the authors decided to design their multicenter cohort to identify predictors of short, intermediate, and long-term ACLR outcomes that would include PROMs, ACL graft failure, and the development of post-traumatic osteoarthritis. The authors aimed to follow this cohort for 10 years, with short and intermediate follow-up data collection at 2 and 6 years after surgery, as the authors knew that certain outcomes of interest, such as the onset of post-traumatic osteoarthritis, would take years rather than months to develop, particularly in a young, athletic population. Like their previous cohort, the authors opted to use PROMs as the primary outcome, as doing so would allow the authors to follow this large cohort of patients over time without necessitating in-person follow-up (and the authors had already invested the time and publications into justifying to the scientific community that PROMs were a valid outcome measure in orthopedic research). However, because they wanted to better understand the relationship between ACLR, preoperative and intra-operative risk factors, and the structural development of post-traumatic osteoarthritis, the authors created a smaller, nested cohort within the larger group that would be followed with longitudinal specialized radiographs, limited use of advanced imaging (MRI), and physical exam-inations, in addition to the PROMs that could be completed remotely. Lastly, because the authors opted to include graft failure as an outcome of interest, they knew that their cohort needed to be large, as ACL revision had occurred only approximately 10% of the time in their previous cohort.

Three obvious questions then arose:

How many patients would we need to enroll, and how many sites/surgeons would that require?

How could the authors collect these preoperative and intraoperative variables reli-ably without overburdening participating surgeons, and in a way that was scien-tifically valid?

How could the authors afford this?

To estimate the size of their cohort, the authors looked to their least likely outcome, which would almost certainly be ACL graft failure, and, given that they wanted to perform multivariable regression modeling with ACL graft failure as the dependent variable, the cohort needed to be large enough to accommodate roughly 15 graft failures per suspected predictor. Thus, to include 15 predictors in their model, the authors would need 225 ACL graft failures, and, given that they observed failure in approximately 10% of their previous cohort, the entire cohort would need to be on the order of 2250 patients.

To enroll such a large number of patients in a timely fashion, the authors aimed to assemble a team of surgeons that, combined, would perform approximately 600 ACLRs per year, allowing the authors to complete enrollment in roughly 4 years. With the VSM-CCF ACLR Registry, the authors demonstrated successful collaboration between 2 institutions, and, with The Ohio State University coming into the fold shortly thereafter, the authors added a third high-volume ACLR center. Through various per-sonal connections and professional relationships, we came to include Hospital for Spe-cial Surgery (Robert Marx), the University of Colorado (Eric McCarty, Michelle Wolcott, and Armando Vidal), the University of Iowa (Ned Amendola and Brian Wolf), and Wash-ington University in St. Louis (Rick Wright, Matthew Matava, and Robert Brophy), as well as additional surgeons at Vanderbilt University (Warren Dunn and John Kuhn), the Cleveland Clinic (Morgan Jones), and The Ohio State University (David Flanigan), bringing the final tally to 17 surgeons at 7 institutions across the country.

With a team of experienced surgeons assembled, the authors' sights turned to creating a system that would allow for accurate but rapid collection of relevant data that could be quickly and easily implemented at the 7 involved institutions. The authors initially utilized a paper-based system that involved data collection forms that could be scanned into a database using optical character recognition software (Teleform, OpenText, Waterloo, Ontario). Creating an electronic data capture system was not realistically possible at this point in time, especially given limited resources. With the help and guidance of their late friend, Dr. Sandy Kirkley, the authors designed a series of standardized PROM questionnaires and surgeon data capture forms. The PROMs were completed by patients prior to their ACLR, and the participating sur-geons captured all of the desired intraoperative variables at the time of the ACLR. From 2004 to 2005, the authors developed an electronic surgeon capture system uti-lizing the Compaq iPAQ, a pocket PC that debuted in April of 2000. Unfortunately, this proved to be an unreliable mechanism after using it for a little over a year, and was later abandoned (returning back to paper forms).

One challenge that the authors encountered while developing their data collection system was getting all surgeons to agree on what and how certain intraoperative variables would be classified. For example, among their intraoperative variables were meniscal tear location, depth, type (degenerative vs acute), and management strategy (repair vs meniscectomy). To demonstrate that their classification scheme, data capture form, and treatment decisions were reliable and reproducible, the authors performed an inter-rater agreement study with video recordings of 18 meniscal tears and asked participating surgeons to classify them accordingly.[21] The authors then duplicated the same strategy to demonstrate agreement in classification of articular cartilage lesions, another important intra-operative variable collected by MOON surgeons.[22]

Yet another hurdle encountered was not how surgeons classified intraoperative variables, but rather how surgeons performed the ACLR itself. Of greatest concern was whether the participating surgeons placed their tibial and femoral tunnels in the same location, as large differences could impact the result of the surgery. Again, the authors performed an intersurgeon and intrasurgeon tunnel variability study utilizing both cadavers and surgical patients to demonstrate that the MOON surgeons placed their tunnels in the same locations, and that the individual surgeons varied little in their tunnel placement from patient to patient.[23,24]

Then the authors needed to overcome possibly one of the most significant hurdles facing a group of 17 senior orthopedic surgeons, their personal preference toward BTB or hamstring autograft. Rather than try to convince those preferring BTB to perform all hamstring autografts or vice versa (which likely would have cost the study multiple surgeons and numerous arguments), the authors performed a systematic review that showed no clinically relevant differences between the 2 choices.[25]

So, the authors had assembled a final team of 17 surgeons at 7 institutions and developed a system that would allow them to collect large amounts of relevant, reliable, and reproducible data in a (relatively) pain-free fashion. The last, and most important, question became how to pay for MOON, especially early on before it received any grant funding.

Consider that MOON carried with it an estimated annual cost of nearly $200,000 at Vanderbilt University alone, and it becomes easy to see why many thought MOON to be impossible. In total, MOON cost nearly $1.4 million to operate between 2001 and 2006, of which none came from National Institute of Arthritis and Musculoskeletal and Skin Disease (NAIMS) grants. The bulk of the early funding was given in the form of unrestricted gifts from Smith & Nephew ($450,000) and Aircast ($200,000), followed by a grant from the National Football League (NFL) Charities ($125,000) and the remainder of the OREF Prospective Clinical Research Grant ($149,000) that the authors had received to cover costs related to following up the VSM-CCF ACLR Registry. The final $450,000 was provided by Vanderbilt University Sports Medicine, generated by an internal tax on partners (Eric McCarty and John Kuhn) and the authors.

Finally, in January of 2002, the authors enrolled the first MOON patient, but the challenges did not stop there. They relied heavily on regular communication to discuss any new and/or ongoing concerns. These were not limited to concerns from the participating surgeons, but also included any issues encountered by the large research support staff that carried out the bulk of the patient enrollment and follow-up, as well as the numerous biostatisticians who helped to make sense of so much data. This was typically done with a group conference call on the second Monday of every month, a call that has taken place nearly every month for the last 15 years. The authors also made it a point to meet in person at least once per year.

By the end of 2005, 3 years into MOON, the authors had enrolled 2340 patients and had followed up with 93% of the cohort by phone and received 85% of PROMs completed at 2 years. Between 2007 and 2008, the group enrolled another 1200 ACLRs that were needed to investigate the impact of meniscus tears and treatment, as well as articular cartilage injuries and treatment on multivariable models.

Although assembling such a large cohort and achieving follow up rates well above 80% represented a huge success and validated the authors' approach, doing so came with significant expense. These costs included a full-time staff of research assistants and coordinators, a project manager, and biostatistician and database support besides coinvestigators with expertise in clinical studies. There were also additional costs associated with the nested cohort, which included training (and retraining) radiology personnel at 3 separate institutions, advanced imaging (MRI), radiographs, blinded evaluations by another surgeon and physical therapist, and more.

Additionally, with such a large (and growing) cohort, from which hundreds of variables were collected from each individual patient, the authors quickly came to a greater appreciation for database design and management. Currently, if one had a Space Shuttle (roughly 122 feet in length) for each data point in the MOON database, the shuttles would span the distance between the surfaces of the earth and the moon (10 million shuttles, covering 1.2 billion feet). What is more astounding is that even with so much data, there has been 98% surgeon compliance (completing intraoperative variable collection), 99% patient participation (agreeing to take part in the study), and 98% completion rates of baseline questionnaires.

By February of 2004, the authors had assembled sufficient preliminary data to apply for a National Institutes of Health (NIH) R01 grant, and they were rejected. The authors subsequently revised their proposal and resubmitted again in November of 2004, only to be rejected a second time. The authors then reorganized our specific aims and objectives and submitted a new NIH grant for the third time in early 2005, and, for the third time, were rejected. However, they were close, and the authors followed the reviewers' critiques and planned a resubmission. Despite having amassed considerable data that demonstrated the worth, validity, and feasibility of MOON, it took a fourth submission before the authors were successfully funded in 2006, a full 15 years after they came to the conclusion that MOON was an answer to their problem. It is worth mentioning again that, at the time (late 2004 to early 2006), the use of PROMs as a primary outcome was a novel concept and a paradigm shift that had not been received with unanimous support by any means.[20] To make their use of PROMs as a primary outcome even more controversial was the gamble that the authors took by adopting 2o PROM questionnaires that, at the time of MOON's inception in 2002, were both less than 4 years old. Despite their early failed attempts to receive federal funding, MOON has successfully renewed its funding on 3 separate occasions to allow for collection of 2-, 6-, and 10-year follow-up data.

The results of MOON and the impact that it has had and will continue to have on ACLR practices nationwide have been discussed elsewhere.[26] Possibly of greater importance than the conclusions drawn from the MOON cohort data is the template that MOON has created for conducting high-quality orthopedic research in the modern age. As a result, MOON has led to several spinoffs including the Multicenter ACL Revision Study (MARS) and MOON Shoulder. Additionally, almost all of the Meniscal Tear and Osteoarthritis Research (MeTeOR) sites were original MOON and/or MARS sites.[27,28]

In closing, the journey to MOON has been a long one, full of ups and downs, successes and failures, and countless lessons learned, but it would have been impossible were it not for the incredible team of surgeons and supporting staff that came together in 2001 (and well before that) to become a part of something bigger than themselves for the betterment of their patients. Now, where will we go next?

REFERENCES

1. Spindler KP, Schils JP, Bergfeld JA, et al. Prospective study of osseous, articular, and meniscal lesions in recent anterior cruciate ligament tears by magnetic resonance imaging and arthroscopy. Am J Sports Med 1993;21(4):551–7.
2. Andersson C, Odensten M, Good L, et al. Surgical or non-surgical treatment of acute rupture of the anterior cruciate ligament. A randomized study with long-term follow-up. J Bone Joint Surg Am 1989;71(7):965–74.
3. Feagin JA, Curl WW. Isolated tear of the anterior cruciate ligament: 5-year follow-up study. Am J Sports Med 1976;4(3):95–100.
4. Kannus P, Järvinen M. Conservatively treated tears of the anterior cruciate ligament. Long-term results. J Bone Joint Surg Am 1987;69(7):1007–12.
5. Odensten M, Lysholm J, Gillquist J. Suture of fresh ruptures of the anterior cruciate ligament. A 5-year follow-up. Acta Orthop Scand 1984;55(3):270–2.
6. Engebretsen L, Benum P, Fasting O, et al. A prospective, randomized study of three surgical techniques for treatment of acute ruptures of the anterior cruciate ligament. Am J Sports Med 1990;18(6):585–90.
7. Hanypsiak BT, Spindler KP, Rothrock CR, et al. Twelve-year follow-up on anterior cruciate ligament reconstruction: long-term outcomes of prospectively studied osseous and articular injuries. Am J Sports Med 2008;36(4):671–7.
8. Buller LT, Best MJ, Baraga MG, et al. Trends in anterior cruciate ligament reconstruction in the United States. Orthop J Sports Med 2015;3(1). 2325967114563664.
9. Spindler KP, Warren TA, Callison JC, et al. Clinical outcome at a minimum of five years after reconstruction of the anterior cruciate ligament. J Bone Joint Surg Am 2005;87(8):1673–9.
10. Bowers AL, Spindler KP, McCarty EC, et al. Height, weight, and BMI predict intra-articular injuries observed during ACL reconstruction: evaluation of 456 cases from a prospective ACL database. Clin J Sport Med 2005;15(1):9–13.
11. Fox JA, Nedeff DD, Bach BR Jr, et al. Anterior cruciate ligament reconstruction with patellar autograft tendon. Clin Orthop 2002;402:53–63.
12. Graham SM, Parker RD. Anterior cruciate ligament reconstruction using hamstring tendon grafts. Clin Orthop 2002;402:64–75.
13. Kaeding CC, Pedroza AD, Parker RD, et al. Intra-articular findings in the reconstructed multiligament-injured knee. Arthroscopy 2005;21(4):424–30.
14. Paul JJ, Spindler KP, Andrish JT, et al. Jumping versus nonjumping anterior cruciate ligament injuries: a comparison of pathology. Clin J Sport Med 2003;13(1):1–5.
15. Piasecki DP, Spindler KP, Warren TA, et al. Intraarticular injuries associated with anterior cruciate ligament tear: findings at ligament reconstruction in high school and recreational athletes. An analysis of sex-based differences. Am J Sports Med 2003;31(4):601–5.
16. Spindler KP, McCarty EC, Warren TA, et al. Prospective comparison of arthroscopic medial meniscal repair technique: inside-out suture versus entirely arthroscopic arrows. Am J Sports Med 2003;31(6):929–34.
17. Irrgang JJ, Anderson AF, Boland AL, et al. Development and validation of the international knee documentation committee subjective knee form. Am J Sports Med 2001;29(5):600–13.
18. Roos EM, Roos HP, Lohmander LS, et al. Knee Injury and Osteoarthritis Outcome Score (KOOS)—development of a self-administered outcome measure. J Orthop Sports Phys Ther 1998;28(2):88–96.

19. Heckman JD. Are validated questionnaires valid? [letter]. J Bone 2006;88(2): 446–52.
20. Zarins B. Are validated questionnaires valid? J Bone Joint Surg Am 2005;87(8): 1671–2.
21. Dunn WR, Wolf BR, Amendola A, et al. Multirater agreement of arthroscopic meniscal lesions. Am J Sports Med 2004;32(8):1937–40.
22. Marx RG, Connor J, Lyman S, et al. Multirater agreement of arthroscopic grading of knee articular cartilage. Am J Sports Med 2005;33(11):1654–7.
23. Wolf BR, Ramme AJ, Britton CL, et al, MOON Knee Group. Anterior cruciate ligament tunnel placement. J Knee Surg 2014;27(4):309–17.
24. Wolf BR, Ramme AJ, Wright RW, et al. Variability in ACL tunnel placement: observational clinical study of surgeon ACL tunnel variability. Am J Sports Med 2013; 41(6):1265–73.
25. Spindler KP, Kuhn JE, Freedman KB, et al. Anterior cruciate ligament reconstruction autograft choice: bone-tendon-bone versus hamstring: does it really matter? A systematic review. Am J Sports Med 2004;32(8):1986–95.
26. Lynch TS, Parker RD, Patel RM, et al. The impact of the Multicenter Orthopaedic Outcomes Network (MOON) research on anterior cruciate ligament reconstruction and orthopaedic practice. J Am Acad Orthop Surg 2015;23(3):154–63.
27. Katz JN, Brophy RH, Chaisson CE, et al. Surgery versus physical therapy for a meniscal tear and osteoarthritis. N Engl J Med 2013;368(18):1675–84.
28. Wright RW, Huston LJ, Haas AK, et al. Effect of graft choice on the outcome of revision anterior cruciate ligament reconstruction in the Multicenter ACL Revision Study (MARS) cohort. Am J Sports Med 2014;42(10):2301–10.

Printed and bound by CPI Group (UK) Ltd, Croydon, CR0 4YY

08/05/2025

01864725-0002